As we rocket into the new century, our toughest challenge lies within ourselves—developing our highest capacities and applying them to empower our lives.

—Joe H. Slate, Ph.D.

WHEN YOU TAP into the healing and rejuvenating power of your mind, the possibilities are limitless. Your personal aura is a life-sustaining energy force that characterizes you as a human being. Understand your aura, and more importantly, utilize it to empower your life, by gaining a deeper understanding of yourself and your place in the cosmos. *Aura Energy for Health, Healing and Balance* brings you the strategies you need to develop your ability to observe, interpret, and affect the aura.

In his latest book, Dr. Joe H. Slate helps you connect with the power to see the aura, interpret it, and fine-tune it. College students have used his techniques to raise grade-point averages, gain admission to graduate programs, and get the jobs they want. Now you can use his aura empowerment program to initiate an exciting new spiral of growth in all areas of your life—mental, physical, and spiritual.

Unleash your internal healing and wellness energies using psychic strategies that balance and attune the mind and body. Fortify your immune system, repair damaged tissue, restore normal organ functions, and slow—in some instances, reverse—aging.

About the Author

Joe H. Slate is a licensed psychologist in private practice and Professor Emeritus at Athens State University. As head of the Psychology Department and Director of Institutional Effectiveness, he established the University's parapsychology research laboratory and introduced parapsychology into the curriculum, a first for the state of Alabama. His research has been funded by the U.S. Army, the Parapsychology Foundation of New York, and numerous private sources. He founded the International Parapsychology Research Foundation which has endowed scholarships programs in perpetuity at both Athens State University and the University of Alabama.

Slate holds a Ph.D. from the University of Alabama, with postdoctoral studies from the University of California. He is Honorary Professor at the University of Montevallo where he participated in the university's curriculum development efforts. He is a member of the American Psychological Association and a Platinum Registrant in the National Register of Health Service Providers in Psychology. He is a frequent lecturer and has appeared on numerous radio and TV programs including Sightings and Strange Universe. His research on the human energy system was recently featured on History TV's *Vampire Mysteries*.

To Write to the Author

If you wish to contact the author, or would like more information about this book, please write to the author in care of Llewellyn Worldwide, and we will forward your request. Both the author and the publisher appreciate hearing from you and learning of your enjoyment of this book and how it has helped you. Llewellyn Worldwide cannot guarantee that every letter written to the author can be answered, but all will be forwarded. Please write to:

Joe H. Slate
c/o Llewellyn Worldwide
2143 Wooddale Drive
Woodbury, MN 55125-2989

Please enclose a self-addressed, stamped envelope for reply, or $1.00 to cover costs. If outside the U.S.A., enclose international postal reply coupon.

AURA
ENERGY
for Health, Healing & Balance

JOE H. SLATE, Ph.D.

Llewellyn Publications
Woodbury, Minnesota

FIRST EDITION
Ninth Printing, 2011

Cover design: Lisa Novak
Book design and editing: Michael Maupin
Photographs courtesy of Joe H. Slate,
  except for pages 25 and 80, by Patricia A. Howell

Library of Congress Cataloging-in-Publication Data
Slate, Joe H.
  Aura energy for health, healing & balance / Joe H. Slate. -- 1st ed.
     p.   cm.
  Includes bibliographical references and index.
  ISBN 13: 978-1-56718-637-6
  ISBN 10: 1-56718-637-8 (trade paper)
  1. Aura.   I. Title.
BF1389.A8S53 1999
133.8'92--dc21   98-46493
                                                    CIP

Llewellyn Publications
A Division of Llewellyn Worldwide Ltd.
2143 Wooddale Drive
Woodbury, MN 55125-2989
www.llewellyn.com
Llewellyn is a registered trademark of Llewellyn Worldwide Ltd.
Printed in the United States of America

Other Books
by Joe H. Slate

Psychic Empowerment

Psychic Empowerment for Health and Fitness

Astral Projection and Psychic Empowerment

Rejuvenation

Psychic Vampires

Beyond Reincarnation

Connecting to the Power of Nature

Psychic Empowerment for Everyone
(with Carl Llewellyn Weschcke)

Astral Projection for Psychic Empowerment
(with Carl Llewellyn Weschcke)

Doors to Past Lives & Future Lives
(with Carl Llewellyn Weschcke)

The Llewellyn Complete Book of Psychic Empowerment
(with Carl Llewellyn Weschcke)

Self Empowerment Through Self Hypnosis
(with Carl Llewellyn Weschcke)

*Self Empowerment Through Self Hypnosis
Meditation CD Companion*
(with Carl Llewellyn Weschcke)

Self-Empowerment and Your Subconscious Mind
(with Carl Llewellyn Weschcke)

Contents

Figures

Author's Note

SEVERAL YEARS AGO, I became faculty adviser to a group of students who were interested in studying psychic phenomena at Athens State University, Alabama (formerly Athens State College). Soon afterward, the International Parapsychology Research Foundation was formed. Within its stated mission of promoting the scientific study of psychic phenomena, the Foundation initiated an endowment drive, introduced parapsychology into the college's instructional program, awarded scholarships, and sponsored scores of laboratory research projects.

To the Foundation, now a private organization, I here express my sincerest appreciation for its commitment to the search for new knowledge, and for its enthusiastic support of my research efforts that have provided the basis for many of the concepts and strategies presented in this book.

I also extend my warmest thanks to the many students who, without stint of time and energy, gave of themselves to my research efforts. I realize that without their help, it would have been impossible for me to have completed this enterprise. Special recognition is due my co-investigators, research assistants, and learned colleagues, all of whom contributed immeasurably to this book. My debt to them is beyond words. Also, to the lecture audiences with whom I shared many parts of this book, I offer my sincerest thanks for their insights and suggestions.

Finally, to the men and women at Llewellyn Publications for their intuitive grasp of my goals for this book from the beginning, I here express my sincerest gratitude.

Writing this book was one of the most rewarding ventures of my life. I hope those who read it will be proportionately rewarded.

Preface

I MAGINE AN ADVANCED energy and information system that contains a true chronicle of your life—past, present, and future. By
referring to it, you could expand your awareness and discover exciting new dimensions to your existence. Imagine further that this system could uncover important resources that would enrich your life
with new insight, growth, and power. Amazing as it may seem, there
exists such a system. It is your personal aura.

The study of the human aura and its empowerment relevance is
at the cutting edge of psychic science today. More than any other
single human trait, the aura manifests the sum and substance of our
existence as an endless life force in the universe. As a developmental
phenomenon, it provides a visible continuum of our evolution from
our earliest beginning. It is an extension of our higher self, and a
manifestation of the cosmic nature of our being. It is the antennae
of consciousness, a treasure-trove of knowledge, and a repository of
limitless growth possibilities. It is a spectacular garment of resplendent beauty that neither fades with age nor unravels with wear. Its

radiance surpasses the brightest works of nature. It has been described by some as the light of God shining out from within us.

The major objective of this book is twofold: to explore the basic nature and makeup of the human aura, and second, to develop relevant strategies to use the aura, not simply as an energy phenomenon, but as our link to the cosmic source of our existence. Perhaps not surprisingly then, our study of the aura is steadfastly empowerment oriented. It stays within the transdisciplinary psychic empowerment perspective, which recognizes the relevance of our dormant potentials and our capacity to tap into them.

This book first examines the essential characteristics of the aura, and then develops strategies for viewing and interpreting the aura as an interactive component of a larger energy system. Next it focuses on intervention strategies designed to empower the aura. Highly specific procedures are introduced to illuminate, attune, energize, and where needed, structurally modify the aura. The book offers innovative, step-by-step strategies for repairing the dysfunctional aura and protecting it against future damage. It develops a wide range of practical empowerment applications—promoting wellness, accelerating learning, breaking unwanted habits, overcoming fear, building self-esteem, increasing creativity, slowing aging, and ensuring career success, to name a few. The book concludes with a seven-day aura empowerment plan designed to initiate a totally new growth spiral.

Admittedly, there are many gaps in our understanding of the human aura, and filling them is a daunting task. While this book attempts the task, it does not claim to have completed it. Nevertheless, it probes with persistence the inexhaustible resources available to us, both within ourselves and the cosmos. It challenges us to reach beyond our limits and discover exciting new dimensions to our existence. It impels us to become *empowered!*

The New Age
of Psychic Empowerment

*The known is finite, the unknown infinite; intellectually we stand
on an islet in the midst of an illimitable ocean of inexplicability.
Our business in every generation is to reclaim a little more land,
to add something to the extent and solidity of our possessions.*

—Thomas Henry Huxley
on the reception of *The Origin of Species* (1887)

I N RECENT YEARS, we have seen a rising interest in the complex
interaction between the mind and body. Many of the empowerment implications of that interaction are now generally acknowledged by conventional science. But often missing from the equation
is the supreme power of the individual to initiate that interaction
and determine its outcome.

The psychic empowerment perspective extends the mind/body
interaction, to include the totality of our existence as mental, physical, and spiritual beings. It emphasizes the continuous mind, body,
and spirit interaction, and our capacity as conscious beings to direct
it. It introduces a totally new paradigm of human existence, and a
whole new world of empowerment possibilities. While recognizing
personal empowerment as the birthright of every human being, it
emphasizes personal responsibility and concern for others. It firmly
holds that we can empower our own lives, and once empowered, we
can help make the planet an empowerment zone for everyone. This
may seem idealistic, but it's what psychic empowerment is all about.

Central to the mind, body, and spirit interaction is the human aura. But understanding the aura, and more importantly, using it to empower our lives, requires a deeper understanding of ourselves and our place in the cosmos. In the following, we will explore our nature as human beings from the psychic empowerment perspective. We will trace the evolution of that perspective and its relevance to our study of the human aura.

Early Beginnings

In its seminal beginnings, the psychic empowerment perspective of human experience centered on investigating two major forms of unexplained phenomena: (1) extrasensory perception (ESP), or conscious awareness occurring independent of sensory experience, and (2) psychokinesis (PK), or the power of the mind to influence matter. Upon establishing the existence of these phenomena, researchers began rethinking the conventional boundaries of human consciousness and developing new perspectives that would make sense of the many emerging yet uncharted territories. The groundwork had been laid for a more holistic, transdisciplinary view of human behavior.

As the psychic empowerment perspective continued to unfold, the focus turned to a careful re-examination of human consciousness and the nature of human existence in the cosmic scheme of things. Emboldened by breakthrough discoveries concerning phenomena such as near-death experiences (NDEs) and out-of-body experiences (OBEs), scientists and philosophers alike began to explore human consciousness and the discarnate realm as sources of power and knowledge. Contributing to that unfolding perspective was the development of more effective procedures for probing the discarnate realm and interacting with higher cosmic planes. The result was an amazing discovery of new sources of power and knowledge. Of profound significance were the breakthrough discoveries that consciousness, including our mental faculties, emotions, and volition, continues undulled in the discarnate dimension. The limitless scope of human existence and, more specifically, the survival of consciousness and personal identity after bodily death were finally confirmed.

Fresh new insight into discarnate survival phenomena gave rise to new assessments of our existence as an indestructible energy force in the universe. Psychic phenomena and the spiritual nature of our being emerged as critical components of a new psychic empowerment perspective that focused on the totality of our existence and new ways of applying psychic knowledge.

At last, the psychic empowerment perspective had turned from superficial speculation to fundamental specification. Highly detailed, laboratory-tested procedures replaced trial-and-error "stab-in-the-dark" approaches whose premises, while creative, were at best unclear. A wide range of practical, step-by-step procedures based on established psychic principles were developed to deliberately access and activate our inner psychic faculties. Laboratory-based procedures were formulated to mentally send and receive thought messages (telepathy), predict the future independently of sensory input (precognition), generate awareness of spatially distant conditions or events (clairvoyance), and influence tangible conditions (PK). Finally available to everyone were new, workable ways of developing psychic potentials and actually applying psychic knowledge, not only to empower our lives individually, but equally as important, to help others and eventually to create global change.

Psychic Empowerment Today

The deluge of the empowering discoveries of psychic phenomena not only challenged conventional wisdom, it opened up a crack that is now a large crevasse. We now know that the psychic dimension of consciousness is a crucial, universal phenomenon. Everyone is psychic with unlimited capacity for growth and self-discovery. In our search for significance and meaning, we must go beyond the physical experience of the material world. The psychic experience breaks the conventional barriers to reveal an exciting new realm filled with endless empowerment possibilities.

Today, the scope of the psychic experience has been expanded to include any event—mental, physical, or spiritual—which either transcends our physical existence or cannot be attributed exclusively to physiological factors. Among the countless examples are psychic healings, discarnate interactions, out-of-body travel, past-life regression, and channeling. It is important to note that such a comprehensive perspective of psychic phenomena, while emphasizing psychical processes, does not exclude biological influences or the effects of certain psychic experiences on biological functions, including those related to better health and fitness.

Although our biological make-up provides the essential condition for our physical survival in this temporal reality, biology alone cannot explain our existence as conscious beings in the universe. We are temporary residents of the planet, but permanent citizens of the cosmos. Biology neither identifies our origin nor designates our destiny. The low road of matter does not lead to the high road of ultimate truth. Non-biological factors, such as a thirst for new knowledge, belief in oneself, a commitment to grow and learn, love for others, and faith are among the powerful influences that define our existence and give meaning to our lives.

A constant theme of the psychic empowerment perspective is the power of the conscious mind. Because it derives from spiritual reality rather than some ultimate meta-level of the brain, human consciousness has primacy over material reality. It is the ground substance of our mental, physical, and spiritual existence. It can initiate new brain functions and deliberately intervene to direct them. It can combine our thoughts, feelings, and emotions to produce new insight and knowledge.

Even so-called autonomic biological functions are subject to the power of the conscious mind. Today, it is generally recognized that uncontrolled negative mental forces such as stress and smoldering hostility can disarm the body, erode our defense systems, lower resistance to disease, and under prolonged circumstances, cause illness or even death. We have, unfortunately, been reluctant to recognize the other side of the coin—the healing and rejuvenating power of the mind. We have known for years that many body organs and systems are highly sensitive to negative psychological factors, but only recently have we developed specific health and fitness strategies based on the positive powers of the mind. Highly detailed psychic strategies that balance and attune the mind and body are now available to literally unleash healing and wellness energies throughout the body. Similarly, rejuvenation strategies that combine mental and physical elements have been developed to decelerate, and in some instances, even reverse aging. Fortifying the body's immune system, repairing damaged tissue, and restoring normal organ functions are not beyond the reach of the empowered mind.

Along a similar line, memory, problem solving, creativity, and mood states are clearly responsive to conscious intervention. Highly specific psychic strategies, based on laboratory research, are now available to improve memory, facilitate problem solving, increase creativity, promote a positive mood state, and even accelerate the rate of learning. These strategies typically recognize the relevance of physiological factors, including the role of bio-chemistry and genetics, but they emphasize the power of the mind to transcend and literally alter specific biological functions, including the fragile circuitry of the central nervous system. To attribute all human behavior to biological factors alone is to deny not only the power of the mind over the body, but also the survival of consciousness and the endurance of intricate mental faculties after death. (For more information on these and related topics, see *Psychic Empowerment* and *Psychic Empowerment for Health and Fitness*.)

Our personal empowerment is primarily a function of choice and self-determination. Rather than being controlled by environment, instinct, or cryptic programming, we are by nature empowered to voluntarily create our own future. We can choose success rather than failure, growth rather than atrophy, and happiness rather than despair. Given the power of choice, we can direct our own lives and pursue our highest goals.

When we tap into the powers of the mind, the possibilities are unlimited. Finding solutions to fractured relationships, acquiring complex physical skills, overcoming fear and anxiety, breaking unwanted habits, building self-esteem, increasing creativity, and accelerating learning are examples of the wide ranging applications of psychic empowerment strategies. Equally as important as these are the potential solutions to devastating global problems such as war, pollution, hunger, and disease that cry out for fresh, creative approaches. Given the recent developments in psychic technology, we can not only enrich our lives, we can make the planet a better place and literally determine its destiny.

In our search for knowledge, each probe of the unknown reveals new possibilities for our personal growth and enlightenment. The signs are encouraging. While often shattering conventional wisdom, newly discovered psychic concepts and techniques are beginning to take hold in a myriad of professional settings—psychotherapy, medicine, criminal justice, industry, and education—with astounding results. Managing pain, accelerating healing, breaking unwanted habits, building self-esteem, overcoming depression, increasing motivation, stimulating creativity, building leadership skills, extinguishing fears, controlling stress, slowing aging, and on a broader scale, promoting cultural change and raising global consciousness are only a few of the diverse applications of psychic knowledge. Every individual and any field of human endeavor can benefit from strategies based on psychic concepts.

Looking Ahead

We have come a long way in our search for psychic knowledge and the development of related empowerment strategies, but the challenges are equally as great today. We are now at the threshold of an exciting new era. New psychic concepts, principles, and technology are constantly emerging. But with each new discovery, we are reminded that becoming personally empowered still requires a commitment to grow, a willingness to explore, and a readiness for change.

Researchers agree that while many phenomena cannot be directly observed, they can nevertheless be inferred, and in many instances, indirectly measured. Still, those deeply hidden realities that do not readily lend themselves to direct observation often escape conventional science. Clear evidence of non-conventional phenomena has been all too often dismissed as either dubious or inconsequential. This book does not hesitate to delve into the deepest, most complex aspects of our existence, to include those phenomena that, for the most part, have either gone unrecognized or else been discounted as irrelevant by conventional science.

In the chapters that follow, we will explore the human aura as a critical component of a complex, interactive energy system. We will probe the nature of the aura and explore its relevance to our existence on this planet. We will uncover the powerful dynamics that underlie our physical, mental, and spiritual interactions. We will develop highly specific, step-by-step strategies designed to stimulate our personal growth and empower us to achieve our highest potentials. Although the concepts and procedures presented in this book may at times seem to explode the conventional wisdom, they steadfastly propel us toward a new level of understanding of ourselves as a permanent, dynamic, empowered life force in the universe.

2

The Aura Energy System

Where the telescope ends, the microscope begins.
Which of the two has the grander view?

—Victor Hugo
Les Misérables (1862)

RATHER THAN AN accidental mixture of cosmic dust, we are by design an unfolding dance of a universal life force. As a conscious, indestructible entity, we exist as an integral component within an infinite energy system. Only through understanding the nature of our existence as a life force entity can we understand the nature of the larger system and the universe as a whole.

Without energy, we would not exist. The human aura is an energy phenomenon within a highly complex system. The aura is the external representation of a creative life force which energizes and sustains our existence. As a functional energy form that envelops the physical body, the aura provides a magnificent channel for interacting with other energy sources and dimensions, including other human aura systems.

From the psychic empowerment perspective, the energies of the aura are believed to emanate from a dynamic energy core situated in the innermost part of our being. That inner core, believed to be located in the body's solar plexus region, is the energy powerhouse

9

that fuels our total being—mental, physical, and spiritual. It is the very essence of our existence—it is our link to the cosmos and our claim to immortality. Together, the aura system, with its powerful inner core and outer aura energies, parallels the larger design of the universe with its cosmic energy core and expansive outer systems. The aura not only signals our uniqueness as a dynamic life force, it provides constant interaction with the higher universal life force as the origin of our being. The psychic empowerment perspective recognizes these two infinite life forces as separate, but with an amazing capacity for oneness.

When the aura and its central core are balanced and attuned to the cosmos, we achieve an empowered state of cosmic congruency with unlimited access to supreme cosmic power. Cosmic congruency is a condition of total oneness in which we experience balance within ourselves and an intimate connection to the universe. It is the key to our mental, physical, and spiritual growth. When we are cosmically congruent, we experience peace and harmony with the highest energies of the universe. Equally as important, we discover totally new growth possibilities within ourselves. A major objective of this book is to develop strategies that bring us into a state of inner and outer oneness in which we have access to the endless powers of the cosmos.

Because the aura mirrors the ultimate energizing force of our existence, discovering its empowering potential is essential to our continued growth. That discovery process must include an understanding of the aura and its relationship to our mental, physical, and spiritual well-being. Given new insight into the aura and its empowering capacities, we can take command of the forces that influence our lives and sweep away the many misconceptions and constrictions that thwart our growth.

The human aura is a unique combination of many characteristics, including but not limited to color, intensity, expansiveness, and structural design. These important features provide a visible representation of our indestructible cosmic make-up, which we call our cosmic genotype. As the counterpart of our biological genotype, our cosmic genotype ensures our individuality as a spiritual entity while endowing each of us with unlimited growth potential. The visible aura gives us an exciting glimpse of our unique cosmic nature and our destiny for permanence as conscious beings in the universe.

Because its origin and make-up are cosmic, the personal aura provides an individualized chronicle of our total existence—past, present, and future. It is a highly sensitive and dynamic force that encodes our divine nature while monitoring our growth and mirroring our strengths and vulnerabilities. Perhaps more importantly, the aura system, when properly used, offers an abundance of new growth possibilities.

The aura system is characterized by continuous change, but within a basically stable structure. An array of internal and external factors constantly interact with the aura to influence its development and functions. As we will see later, biological, environmental, emotional, and social factors, to list a few, can significantly affect the aura. Even conditions and future events unknown to us at the moment can assert a powerful influence on the aura by not only modifying its characteristic coloration and patterns, but altering its energizing capacities too.

Fortunately, the aura has a wondrous capacity for adaptation and renewal. As an integral component of our total growth and development, it tends to spontaneously engage positive influences while repelling negative ones because of the supreme nature of its cosmic origin. By studying the aura and its functions, we can increase our understanding of ourselves and our capacity to use our inner resources to empower our lives.

Following are some of the questions frequently raised about the human aura and its functions.

What is the human aura?

The human aura is a developmental, life-sustaining energy force that characterizes every human being. Without it, we could not exist.

Is the aura always visible?

Under appropriate conditions, which we will discuss in the next chapter, the aura can be seen by almost everyone. Though viewing the aura is often a natural, spontaneous process, refining our aura viewing skills almost always requires some degree of practice using structured procedures. Through practice and experience, we can develop our ability, not only to see the aura, but to interpret it.

Are devices available for viewing the aura?

Although various aids, such as special goggles, are available for aura viewing, they are usually unnecessary, and in some instances, they can actually make viewing more difficult. Various photographic devices, including electrophotography, are also available for recording the aura (or aspects of it), but since the aura is in a state of constant change, these devices are of limited value except as research tools.

Do children see the aura?

The aura is a natural phenomenon, and children with no training in structured viewing procedures often report seeing it. But as we mature, our spontaneous viewing capacities can become suppressed and eventually submerged in the subconscious. It is conceivable, however, that we continue to see the aura and respond to it at a subconscious level throughout our lives.

Will my aura remain unchanged from day to day?

The aura is a dynamic, developmental system that is constantly evolving. Although its unique structure or basic framework is typically stable, the aura system is sufficiently flexible to changes in coloration, intensity, expansiveness, and frequency.

Can I see my own aura?

Highly effective procedures are now available for viewing one's own aura. Several of these procedures are discussed in the next chapter.

How far does the aura extend beyond the physical body?

Although the visible aura, as typically seen, extends from the body only a few inches, the actual aura as an energy phenomenon conceivably extends to infinity. In all probability, the human aura is in constant interaction with other dimensions of time, space, energy, and matter.

Does the environment influence the aura?

The aura is sensitive to the totality of our inner and outer environment. Mental, physical, and spiritual factors constantly interact to influence the aura. Personality traits, health status, personal interests, social factors, emotional states, and surrounding conditions can have an immediate and critical effect on the aura. Even distant global and cosmic events can influence the aura.

What are some of the adverse conditions that affect the aura?

A host of negative mental states such as anxiety, hostility, and frustration assert a wear-and-tear effect on the body and drain the aura system of its energy. Likewise, low self-esteem, a poor self-concept, and negative social interactions can enfeeble the aura and seriously deplete its energy supply. Environmental pollutants and certain drug substances can temporarily discolor or constrict the aura.

What are some of the positive conditions that influence the aura?

Love, the most powerful force in the universe, invariably expands, illuminates, and energizes the aura. Other empowering influences include a positive self-concept, a strong sense of well-being, an inner state of balance and attunement, and a genuine concern for others. Every effort to help others or make the world a better place infuses the aura system with radiant energy.

What is the psychic significance of the aura?

As an individualized chronicle of one's life history, the aura can provide important information not available through other sources. In addition to past-life and present-life experiences, there is mounting evidence to suggest that future events, both positive and negative, can be registered in the aura. Simply viewing the aura can activate our psychic faculties, including telepathy, precognition, and clairvoyance.

Do all auras have color?

The human aura is never without color. Although the intensity and distribution of colors in the aura can vary extensively, the aura is typically characterized by a dominant color within a relatively stable aura structure. While areas of white are sometimes noted in the aura, a totally white aura, which would signify perfection, is non-existent. We will later discuss the significance of aura colors, along with strategies designed to influence them.

Do animals have auras?

Like human beings, all animals have auras, but with characteristics that differ noticeably from human auras. The auras of animals are typically less complex in structure but more intense in coloration than human auras. Compared to animals in the wild, domesticated animals typically have more expansive auras, but with subdued coloration. Interestingly, animal pets often take on certain aura color characteristics, including the dominant coloration of their primary caregivers. With the exception of diseased or distressed animals, including caged animals recently taken from the wild, discoloration is seldom seen in the auras of animals.

Do plants have auras?

Plants, from the smallest to the largest, have their own unique energy systems and are surrounded by an energy field. While that field is typically not called an aura, it has certain characteristics that are similar to human and animal auras. In most instances, the energy patterns around plants appear as an iridescent extension of the plant's basic structure and colors. As we will see in a later chapter, our interactions with plant life, particularly trees, can influence our own energy system.

What is the relationship between the aura and the physical body?

The aura is a visible manifestation of the life force that energizes our total being—mentally, physically, and spiritually. Without that energizing life force, the physical body could not function. Although our physical body depends on the life force as reflected in the aura, the life force does not depend on our physical body. The aura, in manifesting the life force underlying our existence, also manifests our immortality as a spiritual being.

What is the relationship between the aura and the astral body?
The astral body, sometimes called the etheric body, is the non-physical counterpart of the biological body. It is permanently sustained by an energy system of cosmic origin, where the biological body is temporally sustained by that same system. Without that energy source, we could not exist in physical, mental, or spiritual form. As already noted, the human aura is the visible manifestation of that energy source.

What happens to the aura during the out-of-body experience?
During the out-of-body experience, the aura system undergoes marked changes but continues to energize both the physical body and its non-physical counterpart, the astral body. Our energy system, with its energizing core, remains intact but expands its power to accommodate astral travel to distant destinations. It is important to keep in mind that the capacities of our energy system are not limited by tangible realities, including time and space. During the out-of-body experience, we remain an energized entity with power to experience distant dimensions of knowledge and power. Among the most empowering strategies known are those that link us to the supreme cosmic source of our existence.

What is the relationship between the aura and consciousness?
Conscious awareness is the essence of our existence as a permanent energy force. Personal consciousness is cosmic energy uniquely designed to assure both our individuality and our immortality. Our existence as a conscious entity is sustained by an energy system which includes, as already noted, the aura and its inner core. That core is often thought of as the eternal spark of divinity that connects us to our spiritual origins, and gives meaning and permanence to our conscious existence.

What happens to the aura at death?
Death, rather than a termination of our existence as a conscious being, is a gateway to another exciting dimension of continued growth. Although at death the physical body "expires" as a life form,

the non-physical remains energized as it ascends to the discarnate realm. In that realm, the permanent life force reflected in the aura remains the energizing life force underlying our existence as a conscious entity. In some instances, the disengaged aura is seen as a glowing energy form gently rising from the physical body at the time of death.

In summary, the human aura system is intricately connected to our entire being. It permeates and energizes us mentally, physically, and spiritually. It is an ever-evolving chronicle of our lives, from our earliest beginnings to the present. It is the manifestation of our destiny for permanence and greatness. Although its basic structure is relatively fixed, it is always sensitive and responsive to our striving for self-empowerment.

Now equipped with a deeper understanding of the aura and its powerful nature, we are ready to explore exciting new dimensions of the mind, body, and spirit. Our mission—to master new strategies that will empower our lives in the present and prepare us for unlimited growth in the future.

3

How to See the Aura

The eternal mystery of the world
is its comprehensibility.

—Albert Einstein
(1936)

F OR THE MOST part, aura empowerment procedures require literally viewing the aura and identifying its unique characteristics before intervention techniques are applied. Although the aura can often be seen spontaneously, or without deliberate effort, step-by-step strategies for viewing the aura on command and under a variety of circumstances are now available.

In our early laboratory efforts to develop effective aura viewing strategies, whether for viewing one's own aura or that of another person, a major concern was the validity of our procedures. Obviously implied in procedures designed to view the aura is the actual existence of the aura. Could the procedure itself generate false images of a non-existent aura? Is the so-called "visible aura" simply an illusion, a product of suggestion, or figment of the imagination?

To investigate the possibility that structured aura viewing procedures could generate illusions rather than valid perceptions of the aura, we devised a three-phase experiment in which a screen was used during each phase to conceal the subject whose aura was being viewed. The screen, which consisted of ten continuous vertical panels, was of sufficient height to conceal the subject, and of sufficient length to permit easy movement from panel to panel, each of which was numbered, as the hidden subject's aura above the screen was viewed. Five trained aura viewers and ten experimental subjects were used for each phase of the experiment.

In Phase I of the experiment, the viewers independently viewed each subject's aura as the subject stood beside the screen. Once the aura was visible, the subject stepped behind the screen and moved randomly from panel to panel. The viewer's task was to follow the movements of the unseen subject among the numbered panels by viewing the aura extending above the screen. In this phase, all viewers were successful in accurately tracing the subject's movements among the panels.

In Phase II of the study, the subject was positioned behind the screen before the trained aura viewer entered the laboratory. The viewer's first task was to determine the location of the unseen subject behind the screen and then, as in Phase I, to trace the movements of the subject from panel to panel. Although they had not viewed the aura before the subject stepped behind the screen, the viewers were, again without exception, successful in tracing the hidden subject's movements among the numbered panels by viewing the aura above the screen.

Phase III of the study introduced an element of deception into the experiment. The conditions were identical to Phase II, with one exception—no subjects were used for the viewings. Upon entering the laboratory, each viewer was instructed as in Phase II to determine the location of the subject behind the screen and then to trace the subject's movements among the panels, when actually no subject was behind the screen. Without exception, the trained viewers were successful—they saw no auras.

In a replication of this study using other viewers and subjects, the results were the same. Other studies revealed a strong consistency in the aura viewing results obtained for the same individual by multiple independent viewers. Furthermore, photographic recordings of the aura obtained under highly controlled conditions revealed a strong stability in the aura patterns for given individuals over a long period of time. Given these findings, we can conclude with a reasonable degree of confidence that the human aura does indeed exist as an observable reality, and that the procedures designed to view the aura are valid.

In the following discussion, we will explore several aura viewing strategies. As with many other psychic empowerment procedures, a universally favored strategy for viewing the aura has not been forthcoming. Only through practice and experience with many strategies and techniques under a variety of conditions can we discover the approaches that work best for us individually.

Aura Viewing Strategies

For most practice viewing exercises, an off-white background, and natural or indirect lighting are recommended. But once viewing skills are acquired, they can be applied under almost any condition. Some advanced aura specialists report success in viewing the aura even in total darkness, and some prefer moonlight as an ideal viewing condition.

In viewing the aura, it is important to recognize the effects of certain environmental conditions on the aura. Our laboratory studies found that the aura, as a highly sensitive energy phenomenon, is influenced by the time of day, barometric pressure, moon phase, environmental pollutants, and even our clothing. On average, the aura reaches its energized peaks at mid-morning, late afternoon, and early evening hours. Falling barometric pressure tends to slightly reduce the aura's energy supply, where rising barometric pressure tends to replenish it. Almost invariably, a full moon energizes and expands the aura.

Environmental pollutants typically discolor and constrict the aura. Secondhand cigarette smoke is particularly damaging since smoke pollutants are readily absorbed into the aura system and then distributed systematically throughout the physical body. The immediate result is a yellowish brown discoloration in the aura along with severe constriction. It obviously follows that a smoke-free environment not only promotes accurate aura viewing, it is also health-enhancing.

Our studies found that the fabric and color of clothing can dramatically influence the aura's energy patterns. For training purposes, a white cotton or silk robe was found to be the ideal garment worn by the subject during viewing. Some aura specialists claim that the most accurate aura viewing is obtained for the unclothed subject. They often fail to note, however, that any discomfort associated with being disrobed for viewing can adversely influence the visible aura, thus possibly distorting the viewer's conclusions. The experienced viewer will usually discern the impact of apparel on the aura, making disrobing unimportant. We will further examine the effects of various fabrics on the human aura in a later chapter.

A common spin-off effect of aura viewing is the spontaneous activation of the viewer's psychic faculties, including pre-cognition, clairvoyance, and telepathy. Simply viewing the aura seems to call forth relevant psychic information concerning the subject. Many experienced viewers find that they can supplement that spontaneous process by simply quieting the mind and allowing psychic impressions to emerge either within the mind or as projected images in the aura being viewed. For telepathy, visualizing one's own aura interfacing that of the subject to form a thought transfer network is usually effective. For both clairvoyance and precognition, intermittently closing one's eyes and visualizing the subject's aura as a psychic screen upon which relevant information can appear is a useful strategy. Although psychic impressions can emerge instantly as a flash of insight during aura viewing, they often occur in a progressive unfolding of new information.

It is very important to emphasize that aura viewing must never deliberately invade the private world of the subject, whether in casual or structured aura viewing situations. Although viewing the aura is a normal part of person perception for the experienced viewer, and while some information about the subject usually accompanies the process, only by permission do we intentionally probe the subject's inner world of experience.

The White-out Procedure

One of the most effective strategies for viewing the aura is the White-out Procedure. A single trial using this procedure is usually sufficient to bring the aura into full focus. Preceding the actual appearance of the visible aura, the procedure produces an optical illusion, called the white-out effect, which results from expanding the peripheral vision while focusing on the forehead of the subject being viewed. Typically short-lived, the white-out effect is characterized by an expansive, milky-white visual field surrounding the subject. It is almost always accompanied by a mentally passive and deeply relaxed state. Once the illusion disappears, the aura spontaneously comes into view. Attention can then be directly focused on the aura and its specific characteristics, including coloration, structure, magnitude, and design.

For this procedure, either natural daylight or soft, indirect lighting is recommended, with the subject being viewed situated at distances of approximately ten feet from the viewer and approximately two-feet away from an off-white, non-glossy background wall or screen. The four-step procedure as follows requires only a few seconds to bring the aura into view.

Step 1. Physical Relaxation. Give yourself permission to become physically relaxed through a simple, three-step technique called body scan: 1. With your eyes closed, mentally scan your body, beginning at your forehead and progressing downward; 2. Envision a soft glow of relaxation accompanying the scan and eventually enveloping your full body; 3. Silently affirm, *I am now fully relaxed.*

Step 2. White-out. Focus your eyes on your subject's forehead, and slowly expand your peripheral vision to encompass your subject's total surrounding. Once your peripheral vision reaches its limits, allow your eyes to fall slightly out of focus. You will then experience the "white-out effect," a phenomenon in which your subject's surroundings assume a milky-white glow.

Step 3. Focusing. Bring your eyes back into focus, and center your full attention on your subject's forehead. Almost immediately, the aura will come into view.

Step 4. Viewing. You are now ready to view the aura, and focus your attention on its coloration and other characteristics. Should your eyes tire during viewing, close them for a few moments or look briefly into the distance away from your subject. If the aura begins to fade at any point during viewing, close your eyes briefly and then repeat the procedure.

Aside from its usefulness in aura viewing, the white-out technique, when modified, can be used in hypnosis as an induction procedure. For that application, a shiny object, such as a brass tack positioned on the ceiling above the reclining subject, provides a convenient point of focus. Following a brief period of relaxation, the hypnosis subject focuses on the tack, then slowly expands peripheral vision to induce the white-out effect. Once white-out has occurred, the eyes are closed as suggestions of depth and drowsiness are presented. Other selected deepening techniques, such as reverse counting and appropriate imagery, can then be applied to deepen the trance state to the desired level.

Our discussion of the white-out technique would be incomplete without considering its application as an investigative tool in discarnate survival research. On the surface, that use of the technique may seem rather farfetched. But if our existence as a life-force entity continues in the discarnate dimension, then probing that dimension through aura viewing strategies assumes greater relevance, and in fact, becomes a plausible investigative option.

Discarnate survival phenomena can be explained as a merging process in which two or more energy dimensions interface or interact. Whether spontaneous or induced, discarnate phenomena are always purposeful and potentially empowering. Simply experiencing discarnate manifestations can be enlightening because they affirm our survival as a conscious entity with identity intact following our transition to the other side. Of even greater importance, discarnate interactions can open totally new channels of personal growth and fulfillment.

As a strategy for researching discarnate manifestations, especially in settings with a long history of sightings, the white-out technique, when appropriately applied, can literally bring discarnate energy manifestation into full view, a phenomenon called interdimensional materialization. Although it departs considerably from our topic of aura viewing strategies, the account that follows is considered relevant to our discussion because it explores, albeit in considerable detail, the effectiveness of the white-out technique in probing other dimensions with aura-like energy manifestations.

The innovative application of the white-out technique as an interdimensional materialization tool was illustrated by a group of forty students enrolled in an experimental parapsychology course at Athens State College (now Athens State University) in Alabama. The course activities included investigating a legend concerning the recurring campus apparition of a young woman who was often seen keeping her late night vigil from a third floor window of McCandless Hall, a Greek Revival structure that houses the school's art, music, and drama programs. The legend claims that a beautiful young actress, whose stage name was Abigail, performed at the hall's auditorium in the opera *La Traviata* shortly after the building's construction near the turn of the twentieth century. Following her brilliant performance, the young actress, dressed in a white gown and clutching a bouquet of red roses, made her final curtain call before an enthralled audience, and in an emotional farewell, vowed to return. She later departed with the opera troupe into the blustery night for the long carriage ride to her next engagement.

As the legend goes, her journey was tragically cut short. Around midnight, the caravan was caught in a severe thunderstorm. Her horse-drawn carriage, vibrating against the unrelenting force of wind and torrential rain, bounced and swayed from side to side. Flashes of lightning gave only brief glances of the treacherous road ahead. Upon approaching a narrow bridge, the horses, startled by a sudden flash of lightning and crash of thunder, lunged forward, disengaging the carriage. The carriage, racing out of control, hurled over the bridge, crashing onto the bedrock below. The actress, mortally wounded, was pulled from the tangled wreckage. Still wearing the white gown and clutching the bouquet of red roses, she whispered her final words, "I have a promise to keep. I must return."

Deep into the winter months following her death, a ghostly image of a willowy young woman, her golden hair glistening in the moonlight, was seen standing at a third-floor window of McCandless Hall. Arrayed in white and clutching a bouquet of red roses at her breast, she appeared only briefly before fading into the darkness. Through the years, the sightings continued—a beautiful but pensive young woman bathed in radiant light, faithfully keeping her late night vigil.

Upon completing a background investigation of the recurring apparition, the parapsychology class assembled around midnight in the third floor art studio of McCandless Hall where the image of the young woman had been frequently sighted. After a brief period of quiet meditation, several students in the group collectively witnessed the gossamer apparition—a beautiful young woman standing in the shadows near a window. The remaining students were then instructed to used the white-out technique in an effort to bring the apparition into view. With the window as their focal point, they expanded their peripheral vision to take in as much of the room as possible, whereupon the apparition of Abigail, still standing near the window, became immediately visible to all of the forty students.

The interaction that followed confirmed many of the legend's details, while providing some interesting additional information. As it turned out, the actress's promise to return was motivated by more than her attachment to the townspeople. Communicating with the group through table tilting, a technique in which a light table taps out answers to questions posed by the group, she admitted having fallen in love with the town's young attorney. During her brief visit to the town, they had met secretly in the art studio, where following her death, she intermittently returned for almost a century. As the session neared conclusion, the group explored with Abigail the growth opportunities available in the discarnate realm, after which the glowing apparition slowly faded from sight.

After the session, Abigail was popularized by the media, including the national tabloids. Accounts of the legend appeared in journals and even a college textbook. Over the years, she became the topic of numerous research efforts, some of them rather ineptly designed expressly to disprove the legend and thus erase it from history. But as if to challenge more noble explorations of the unknown, the apparition continued to appear, always in the late evening hours, and in particular on November 12, the apparent anniversary of her death. Even today, a new student or campus guest, totally unfamiliar with the legend, will report seeing the glowing image of a beautiful young woman, her golden hair glistening in the moonlight, keeping her late night vigil from a third-floor window of McCandless Hall.

As a footnote, a tree reportedly planted in Abigail's memory shortly after her untimely death stands a few feet from the stage entrance of McCandless Auditorium (Figure 1). Now a giant beech, the tree remains a tangible testament of a small town's enduring love for the talented actress, and a silent reminder that, after all is said and done, you cannot kill a legend.

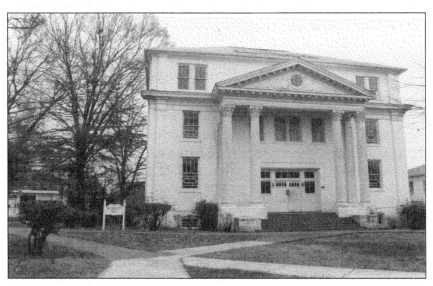

FIGURE 1. MCCANDLESS HALL, ATHENS STATE UNIVERSITY. The apparition of a young woman believed to be Abigail can still be seen at a third-floor window of this stately hall. According to legend, the beech tree at the left of the building was planted in her honor soon after her death near the turn of the twentieth century *(Photo by Patricia A. Howell)*.

The effectiveness of the white-out technique in probing the discarnate realm as well as viewing the human aura suggests a common cosmic energy source and similarity in the underlying dynamics of these two energy phenomena. The white-out technique seems to pull back the cosmic curtain to reveal exciting new dimensions of energy. Although it may undergo transformation, transition, and change, cosmic energy is never lost. From the psychic empowerment perspective, discarnate phenomena, like the aura itself, are meaningful energy manifestations of the highest cosmic order. Our probes into these phenomena can reveal important knowledge concerning the nature of our present existence and our destiny, not simply for survival, but for endless growth.

Perhaps not surprisingly, the white-out technique, as well as other aura viewing procedures, can be applied to monitor changes in the aura associated with the out-of-body experience and other altered states of consciousness. These applications usually require viewing the aura immediate before, during, and after the experience. We will later explore the influence of various altered states on the human aura.

The Focal-Point Procedure

The Focal-point Procedure requires conditions very similar to those of the White-out Procedure. This viewing strategy is especially recommended for individuals who experience difficulty seeing color in the aura. Natural or soft, indirect lighting is recommended. Here is the procedure:

> **Step 1. Preliminaries.** Position your subject at a distance of approximately two feet away from an off-white, non-glossy background screen. On the background screen, place a small shiny object, such as a thumbtack, adhesive dot, or star, a few inches to the upper left or right of your subject. The shiny object must be big enough to be seen clearly from a distance of at least ten feet.

> **Step 2. Relaxation.** At a viewing distance of approximately ten feet from your subject, close your eyes, take in a few deep breaths, and clear your mind of all active thought.

Step 3. Gazing. After a few moments of relaxation, gaze at the shiny object positioned on the screen behind your subject. Continue gazing at the object until a whitish glow appears around your subject, typically within a few seconds. Keep your attention on the shiny object until the whitish glow around your subject assumes coloration.

Step 4. Aura Viewing. Once you see color in the aura, shift your attention from the shiny object directly to the aura, and observe its various characteristics. Should the aura begin to fade away at any time during viewing, return your focus to the shiny object and repeat the procedure. If your eyes tire during the procedure, close them briefly or look into the distance for a few moments and then resume viewing.

The Triangle Erector Procedure

The Triangle Erector Procedure is one the most highly preferred aura viewing strategies because of its effectiveness in not only bringing the full aura into view but also stimulating positive interactions between the viewer and subject. Subjects being viewed by this procedure usually appear more relaxed and responsive than when viewed by other methods, possibly because the procedure does not require prolonged gazing at either the subject or a single background point. The procedure uses eye movements among three designated points on a background screen to mentally erect a triangle, whereupon the aura comes into view, first around the subject's head and shoulders, and then around the full body.

The physical arrangement for the Triangle Erector Procedure is similar to that of other aura viewing strategies. Soft, indirect lighting and an off-white, non-glossy background screen are recommended. Here is the procedure:

Step 1. Preliminaries. With the subject positioned approximately two feet from the background screen, designate the three points of a triangle by placing adhesive dots on the screen. One dot is placed a few inches above the subject, and two dots are placed at waist level, with one to each side of the subject at a few inches from the body.

Step 2. Pre-viewing Conditioning. At a viewing distance of approximately ten feet from your subject, conduct a body scan by closing your eyes for a few moments and mentally scanning your body from the head downward, releasing all tension as you go.

Step 3. Triangle Erector Exercise. Open your eyes and focus your full attention on the dot above your subject's head. After a brief moment of gazing at that point, shift your attention to the dot situated at your subject's lower left. Gaze at that point for a few moments, and then shift your attention to the dot at your subject's lower right. Following a brief moment of gazing at that point, complete the triangle by shifting your attention to the starting point—the dot above your subject. Continue gazing at that point until the aura comes into view, typically within a few seconds. Note: For some viewers, the aura will become visible early-on in the erector exercise.

Step 4. Aura Viewing. Shift your gaze from the dot above your subject and focus your attention directly on the aura. Note specific aura characteristics or areas of particular interest or activity. Should the aura begin to fade at any time during viewing, focus your attention on the dot above your subject and repeat the triangle erector exercise.

Step 5. Psychic Responsiveness. Note the psychic impressions, particularly clairvoyance, that often accompany this procedure.

Many of our aura viewers found that with practice of this viewing strategy, they could effectively substitute imaginary points for adhesive dots on the background screen.

Prior to our development of the Triangle Erector Procedure for aura viewing, our studies found that simply closing the eyes and erecting a mental triangle through eye movement can stimulate the third eye, a faculty which is associated with clairvoyance and remote viewing. In the experimental setting, research subjects more than doubled the accuracy of their performance on clairvoyance and remote viewing tasks when the mental triangle technique was introduced. Our studies further suggested that activating the third eye faculty through this mental technique produced a "chaining effect," in which both telepathy and precognition were chained together and stimulated. Our later studies found that the psychic performance levels significantly increased for our experimental subjects following practice in aura viewing using the Triangle Erector Procedure. Because of its apparent psychic stimulating and chaining effects, the Triangle Erector Procedure is considered an excellent psychic development tool.

The Hand Triangle Procedure

The Hand Triangle Procedure is another highly efficient strategy for both viewing the aura and generating relevant psychic impressions concerning the subject, especially precognition. A major advantage of this procedure is that it can be implemented under generally non-structured viewing conditions, and at wide-ranging distances from the subject. Here is the procedure:

Step 1. Triangle Formation. Form a triangle with your hands by first bringing together the tips of your thumbs to form the base of the triangle. Then bring the tips of your index fingers together to form the top of the triangle.

Step 2. Frame Adjustment. Use the triangle as a frame within which to view your subject. Adjust the frame by moving your hands in and out until you find the distance which provides the ideal space within the triangle for viewing your subject.

Step 3. Aura Viewing. Observe your subject through the triangle until the aura appears, typically within seconds. Remove the triangle by slowly separating and then relaxing your hands. You can now view the aura in its fullness or focus on particular characteristics or areas of activity. Should the aura begin to fade, repeat the procedure.

Step 4. Psychic Responsiveness. Note the psychic impressions, particularly precognition, that often emerge spontaneously during the viewing process.

The Walk-in Procedure

The aura is a highly expansive energy phenomenon. It encircles the body and radiates in all directions, forming concentric zones of energy with specific rims or perimeters as borders for energy regions of varying intensities. As the energy zones extend beyond the physical body and its energizing core, they typically decrease progressively in intensity, with the zone nearest the physical body showing the greatest concentration of energy. Because of the energy diffusion process, the outer regions of the aura are invisible to the naked eye of even the most skilled aura viewer.

Although a total of seven external energy zones are believed to typify the human aura, the abounding diffusion of outer aura energy is probably limitless. Strategies designed to explore the various zones and their borders suggest that the outermost region, unlike the inner zones, has no outer rim, thus possibly extending to infinity.

The Walk-in Procedure is an interactive aura viewing strategy that progressively guides the viewer into the subject's energy zones until the aura becomes visible. The procedure recognizes the existence of numerous concentric aura zones encircling an individual as well as the diminishing intensity of those zones as they extend away from the physical body. As the viewer deliberately "walks into" the energy field of the subject, interaction between the two aura systems tends to occur, with the subject's outer, more diffuse aura zones helping the viewer's efforts to see the more intense zones situated nearer to the subject's physical body.

For this viewing procedure, either natural daylight or subdued, indirect lighting is recommended with the subject whose aura is being viewed situated approximately two feet from an off-white background screen. Here is the procedure:

Step 1. Aura Field Interaction. Assume a viewing distance of approximately twenty feet from your subject. At that distance, you are probably within your subject's noticeable energy field. Briefly close your eyes and note any impressions of the energy interaction between your own energy field and that of your subject.

Step 2. The First Approach. View your subject, and slowly take three or four steps forward as you note changes in the energy interactions. While focusing on your subject, particularly the head and shoulder region, note any visible manifestations of the aura, such as coloration or brightness.

Step 3. Additional Approaches. Repeat Step 2 until the aura comes clearly into view. Once the aura becomes visible, it may be necessary to adjust your focus by moving a few steps forward or backward until you achieve your ideal viewing distance.

Step 4. Aura Viewing. Once you have determined your ideal viewing distance, focus your attention of the aura and its various characteristics.

This procedure can be compared to the stereoscope or magic eye technique which requires adjusting the distance of the object being viewed in order to reach the ideal, three-dimensional viewing distance. For the typical aura viewer, the ideal viewing distance for the human aura ranges from approximately eight to twelve feet. That distance, however, can vary significantly among viewers. Even in replicated viewings of the same subject, the ideal viewing distance will vary from viewing to viewing. These variations are probably due to a host of factors, including the current mental and physical states of the viewer and the subject, as well as the surrounding viewing conditions.

As we will discover in a later chapter, the zones of aura energy and their relative strengths can be assessed through a strategy using a pair of metal dowsing rods. The rims of each zone, with the exception of the most distant zone which appears to radiate endlessly, can be identified, and a map of aura zones can be constructed. The map, using an appropriate distance scale, can provide a comprehensive picture of the concentric zones and their characteristics. The application of dowsing rods in identifying areas of aura dysfunction is also discussed in a later chapter.

Because of the aura system's extensive energy field along with its capacity to generate and disperse energy, it should not be surprising to find that concentrations of energy can be deliberately formed and transferred to selected targets, including other aura systems at considerable spatial distances. Examples of this intervention phenomenon, which we will later explore, are the numerous instances of psychic healing that appear to involve the literal transfer of healing energy from the healer's aura system to that of the recipient.

The Psychic Perception Procedure

The aura viewing procedures we have discussed to this point emphasized strategies that use visual perception. We have explored procedures structured specifically to adapt our vision mechanisms to the energies of the aura system so that the aura becomes visible to the human eye. We have noted that a frequent side benefit of these procedures is the activation of our psychic faculties, once the aura is visible. We discovered that simply viewing the aura is an excellent way to exercise our psychic faculties and gain important information unavailable to us through other channels. Even repressed experiences or impulses buried deeply in the subject's subconscious are often evident during aura viewing.

While viewing the aura can activate our psychic capacities, we can also use our psychic faculties to view the aura. The Psychic Perception Procedure is a viewing strategy specifically designed to make aura viewing independent of sensory perception. This somewhat subjective procedure relies on our psychic capacity, not only to view the aura but to determine its psychic relevance. Many skilled aura viewers use this procedure in conjunction with other more direct viewing strategies because of its capacity to bring forth additional, highly relevant information.

Because the procedure is relatively unstructured, it can be used in a variety of situations. It requires that we are within the subject's energy field, but not necessarily in close proximity to the subject. At distances of more than about twenty feet from the subject, the technique has questionable usefulness except for the highly experienced aura specialist.

Many gifted psychics deliberately use this procedure during their psychic readings because of its spontaneity and non-invasive nature. Rather than actively probing the subject's innermost thoughts or emotions, it psychically envisions the external energy manifestations which, like many of our other physical features, are always present for others to see and respond to. Here is the procedure:

Step 1. Psychic Receptivity. With your eyes closed, generate a state of psychic responsiveness by actively sensing your subject's aura energies, paying particular attention to characteristics such as intensity, frequency, and positive or negative valence as they interface your own aura system.

Step 2. Energy Interaction. Sense the interaction of your energies with those of your subject. Specifically note unusual activity, such as turbulence, imbalance, or weakness in your subject's energy field.

Step 3. Pattern Imagery. Allow images of energy patterns, including such irregularities as breaks or tears in the aura, to accompany the energy interaction. Form an overall mental picture of the aura's energy patterns.

Step 4. Color Imagery. Allow images of the aura's color make-up to emerge. Sense the incoming frequencies and their color characteristics. Your psychic mind has the amazing capacity to sort aura energy frequencies into their appropriate color categories.

Step 5. The Total Aura. Combine your impressions of energy patterns and color characteristics to form a mental picture of your subject's total aura. Pay particular attention to the psychic impressions that accompany this process.

Once you have completed this procedure for psychically viewing the aura, you may wish to literally view your subject's aura, using any of the more objective procedures previously discussed, to validate your psychic perceptions.

Some highly skilled aura viewers use an adaptation of this procedure to remotely view the auras of their subjects from great distances, including by phone or Internet. If indeed the energies of the aura extend into infinity, it would follow that spatial distance would not necessarily deter aura interactions. It would seem plausible, however, that only the highly sensitive and experienced aura specialist would experience the interaction and psychically perceive the aura from great distances.

The Subliminal Perception Technique

A variation of the Psychic Perception Procedure is the Subliminal Perception Technique. This technique is based on the premise that we perceive and respond to certain stimuli, including the human aura, at levels below our conscious thresholds for perception, a phenomenon called subliminal perception. Unlike psychic perception, subliminal perception requires sensory stimulation, which is then perceived and interpreted subconsciously. As applied to the human aura, this perspective holds that we physiologically sense the aura but perceive and respond to it only at the subconscious level. Although subliminal perception is a function of the subconscious, it can assert a powerful influence on our conscious perceptions and behaviors. The goal of the Subliminal Perception Technique is to bring our subconscious perceptions of the aura into conscious awareness.

Supportive of subliminal perception as it relates to the aura is the so-called "chemistry" or "connection" which we often experience in our relationships with individuals and groups. Although these phenomena could be explained as the literal interactions of two aura systems, they may also result from our subconscious perceptions of the auras of persons with whom we interact. Only when we become aware of our subconscious perceptions can we explain many of our behaviors toward others.

Further supporting the relevance of subliminal perception in viewing the aura are our responses to inorganic—albeit excellent—representations of living objects, such as those seen in artificial plants or lifelike animal models. Although many of these lifeless objects are convincingly lifelike, we perceive them differently, possibly because of the missing aura. Similarly, excellent sculpted human figures, such as wax figures of famous persons, can be lifelike in every visible detail, but we perceive them as lifeless because of the missing aura. If we could develop the technology required to imbue an artificial figure with aura-like energies, the figure could conceivably assume a totally lifelike appearance. Among the possibilities are strategies similar to those used in electrophotography. By electrically generating a light-emitting transference of electrical charge around the figure to produce a corona discharge (as in electrophotography), we could possibly simulate the aura and imbue the sculpted figure with truly convincing lifelike qualities. The same procedure could be used with other models of life forms, including the models of prehistoric plants and animals found in museums, to enhance their lifelike characteristics.

The Subliminal Perception Technique is designed primarily to bring subliminal perceptions of the aura into conscious awareness. The technique holds that our subconscious perceptions of the aura influence our impressions and interactions with the subject. By uncovering these subliminal influences, we can increase our understanding of the subject and assume greater command of our subconscious processes, including our hidden psychic faculties.

The Subliminal Perception Technique differs significantly from other aura viewing procedures in that it does not require the physical presence of a subject. Through imagery of the subject, it can retrieve relevant past perceptions stored in the subconscious as well as important psychic impressions being currently registered there. This strategy, like the Psychic Perception Procedure, usually produces information beyond that available through the more direct viewing strategies. Here is the procedure:

Step 1. Mental Imagery. With your eyes closed, envision your subject in as much detail as possible. As images take shape in your mind, focus on your subject's specific physical characteristics. Reflect on your most recent interaction with your subject.

Step 2. Aura Perception. As you continue to envision your subject, allow the aura to form spontaneously around the image in your mind. Take adequate time for the full aura to become visible, then focus on its specific characteristics, including coloration, expansiveness, unique patterns, and other distinguishing features. Sense your responses to your subject's aura as it takes shape in your mind.

Step 3. Psychic Perception. Give special attention to the psychic impressions accompanying the imagery process. Spontaneously allow relevant past, present, and future information concerning your subject to come forth. Mentally affirm: *The abundant resources of my innermost being, both conscious and subconscious, are now available to me.*

Step 4. Conclusion. End the procedure by reviewing your conclusions and exploring ways of using them. If your subject is physically present, validate your conclusions by viewing the aura using any of the direct viewing strategies previously discussed.

The Subliminal Perception Procedure can be used to explore interpersonal relationships and promote more positive interactions, particularly with significant others. It can produce relevant information that explains our interactions and empowers us to productively manage our relationships. Couples using this procedure often find that they better understand each other, and are more sensitive to each other's needs. The exercise can also promote more positive interactions between parent and child, especially in the adolescent years during which rapid change usually occurs in the relationship. In the work setting, the procedure can uncover better strategies for shaping positive relationships, particularly with difficult people.

More research is needed to explore in greater depth the complex nature of subliminal perception, and to develop empowerment strategies that use this powerful phenomenon.

Viewing Your Own Aura

A major challenge in our study of the human aura is the mastery of reliable strategies for viewing not only the aura of others, but our own aura, too. Although several promising self-viewing strategies have been developed in recent years, they are often speculative in nature and their effectiveness has not always been adequately demonstrated. Our studies found that self-viewing efforts using a mirror and other surfaces, including water, dark glass, and various polished metals, are generally unsuccessful in accurately reflecting aura energies. Although these surfaces can, under certain conditions, generate impressions of the aura, the images are usually a far cry from the actual aura. With a few rare exceptions, conventional photography has likewise failed to accurately capture the aura. Experimental efforts to record the aura using certain advanced video and photographic technology have shown promise, but more research is needed to validate these innovative techniques and determine their reliability.

Even with the most advanced aura viewing strategies, our self-viewing efforts are, by nature, limited. They are obviously subjective, and they typically provide only a partial, close-up view of the aura. Psychologically, we tend to experience the totality of ourselves rather than specific parts that we isolate for self-inspection and analysis. Furthermore, our past experiences, interests, attitudes, preferences, and biases can influence our perceptions, particularly of ourselves. Awareness of these tendencies and their influences will promote greater accuracy in our aura self-viewing efforts.

Among the other potential problems with aura self-viewing is the spatial distance normally required for direct aura viewing. Since we cannot view our own aura in its totality from outside our own body, except possibly during the out-of-body experience, spatial distance becomes a major consideration in our self-viewing efforts. Viewing strategies requiring considerable physical distance between the subject and the viewer have little or no applicability to self-viewing.

Fortunately, the distance generated by extending the hand is usually sufficient for at least limited aura viewing. It is not surprising, then, that hand-viewing strategies have emerged as among the most effective and convenient approaches for aura self-viewing. Generally, the characteristics of the aura surrounding the hand, particularly coloration and magnitude, are fairly representative of the total aura.

The Aura Hand-viewing Procedure

The Aura Hand-viewing Procedure is designed to help self-viewing of the aura surrounding the hand and lower arm. Like other aura-viewing strategies, this procedure requires natural or indirect lighting and an off-white background. Here is the procedure:

Step 1. Relaxation. Let yourself become relaxed by taking in a few deep breaths and exhaling slowly as you clear your mind of all active thought.

Step 2. Finger Spread. Extend your hand, and hold it at arm's length with your fingers slightly spread against an off-white background.

Step 3. Visualization. Visualize a small dot floating in the space between your thumb and index finger.

Step 4. Fixed Gazing. Fixedly gaze at the imaginary dot until the aura appears, usually within seconds, first around your thumb and right index finger, then around your full hand and lower arm.

Step 5. Aura Viewing. Once the aura is clearly visible, shift your gaze directly to it, and observe its characteristics.

NOTE: Should you tire at any point in the exercise, take a few moments to relax, and then resume the procedure.

The Finger-Count Procedure

A variation of the Aura Hand-viewing Procedure is the Finger-count Procedure. This strategy requires counting the fingers of the outstretched hand as it is held against an off-white background. Here is the procedure:

Step 1. Finger Count. With your hand outstretched and held with the fingers spread apart, slowly count your fingers one-by-one beginning with the thumb. Gaze briefly at the tip of each finger as you count it.

Step 2. Reverse Finger Count. As your hand remains outstretched and your fingers spread apart, reverse the counting procedure by slowing counting your fingers backward from five to one, beginning with the little finger and ending with the thumb. As in Step 1, gaze briefly at the tip of each finger as you count it.

Step 3. Finger Gaze. Gaze at the tip of your middle finger for a few moments, then expand your peripheral vision to include your full hand. Almost immediately, a soft white glow will appear around your hand, followed by the colorful aura.

Step 4. Aura Viewing. With the aura now in view, you can shift your attention directly to it and observe its features in detail.

The Hand Triangle Procedure
(Adapted for Self-viewing)

The Hand Triangle Procedure as previously discussed can be readily adapted to self-viewing. When used to view one's own aura, the procedure retains its dual role of bringing the aura into view and activating our psychic faculties. The procedure requires natural or soft, indirect lighting and an off-white background screen. Here is the procedure:

Step 1. Triangle Formation. With your hands held at arm's length a short distance from the background screen, erect a triangle by first bringing together the tips of your thumbs to form the base of the triangle. Then bring the tips of your index fingers together to form the top of the triangle.

Step 2. Visualization. While viewing the triangle against the off-white screen, visualize a small dot at the center of the triangle and focus your full attention on the imaginary dot.

Step 3. Fixed Gazing. Fix your gaze on the imaginary dot and continue gazing at it until the aura appears, typically within seconds, first inside the triangle and then around your hands and lower arms.

Step 4. Aura Viewing. Once the aura is visible, note its coloration, expansiveness, and other distinguishing features.

Step 5. Psychic Activation. To activate your psychic faculties, focus your full attention on the concentration of energy in the triangle formed by your hands as you allow psychic insight to unfold.

Step 6. Empowerment Affirmations. Conclude the procedure by affirming your power to view your own aura and use your aura energies as channels for psychic growth.

This self-viewing procedure is one of the most powerful strategies known for activating one's psychic faculties. Our experimental subjects found that by simply focusing on the aura energies that formed in the triangle at Step 4, they could effectively open their telepathic sending and receiving channels. Also, precognitive and clairvoyant impressions almost always accompanied this stage of the procedure. In our studies of remote viewing, we found that the triangle could serve as a frame in which psychic images of distant realities could be clearly depicted. This adaptation was particularly effective for our subjects who experienced only marginal success with other ESP procedures.

The Palm-Motion Procedure

The human aura system is consistently responsive to our efforts to stimulate and intensify its energy capacities. The Palm-motion Procedure is an aura self-viewing strategy designed to generate a transient but highly visible concentration of energy in the hands. The procedure requires only a few seconds and few controls other than an off-white background and soft lighting to help with color perception.

Step 1. Palm Contact. Bring the palms of your hands together lightly, and gently rub them against each other in first circular and then to-and-fro motions. You will notice almost immediately the build-up of warm energy in your palms.

Step 2. Palm Separation. With the palms of your hands remaining together, reach forward, and at arm's length, slowly separate your hands to create a narrow space between them. You will immediately notice a mild tingling in your palms and fingertips.

Step 3. Energy Perception. Center your attention on the narrow space between your hands, and note the whitish glow. Adjust the distance between your hands until color appears.

Step 4. Cupped Palms. With your hands still held at arm's length, gently cup your hands to create some distance between your palms while maintaining the narrow space between your fingertips.

Step 5. Energy Channel. After focusing for a few moments on the space between your fingertips, bring your fingertips together, and then slowly separate them. You will immediately see a channel of glowing energy between your fingertips. Adjust the distance between your fingertips until you notice the appearance of color, which typically matches that of the color seen in the space between your hands in Step 3 above.

Step 6. Aura Viewing. Gaze at your cupped hands still facing each other until the aura appears around them, then turn your hands so that you face your palms. Note the enveloping aura and its various characteristics.

In Step 6 of this procedure, a ball of iridescent energy can often be seen gathering in the cupped hands. Many psychic healers use an adaptation this procedure immediately prior to healing to generate a concentration of positive energy that they, in turn, transfer to the subject as healing energy by turning their palms toward the recipient and in some instances, gently massaging the aura.

The Palm-viewing Procedure has shown interesting promise as a psychokinesis (PK) strategy. In our laboratory, a group of experimental subjects used the procedure to induce motion in a pendulum object suspended under a bell jar. For this exercise, five subjects, who were seated at a distance of approximately six feet from the jar, used the procedure to generate a concentration of energy and target it toward the pendulum. Once the channel of glowing energy became visible between the fingertips in Step 5 of the procedure, they pointed their fingers, with palm sides down, toward the pendulum and mentally commanded it to move. Almost instantly, the pendulum responded, first with a slow turning motion and then with distinct swinging motions until it struck the sides of the jar.

On a broader scale, the Palm-viewing Procedure can be used as a strategy for infusing the planet with positive energy. Once the concentration of energy is formed in your palms, your hands are turned palm sides forward to disperse radiant energy either as a band of light around the planet, or as a body of light fully enveloping the planet. For this application of the procedure, a globe can be introduced to help the sending process. This adaptation is particularly effective in group settings, with the globe, as a tangible representation of the earth, placed at the center of the group. While facing the globe, the group generates positive energy and then, with palms turned toward the globe, disperses it in the form of light around the world. The procedure is usually concluded with affirmations of peace and love.

The Psychic Self-Perception Procedure

From the psychic empowerment perspective, knowledge alone is empowering, but the ultimate power of knowledge rests in its personal relevance. It follows that merely expanding our awareness of the aura is empowering, but if we could connect that awareness to our innermost self, it would become even more forceful. The Psychic Self-perception Procedure, a modification of the Psychic Perception Procedure previously presented, is designed to accomplish that goal.

The capacity to perceive oneself and contemplate the meaning of one's existence is universal, traditionally considered a uniquely human trait. Admittedly, many lower animals acquire highly complex behavioral patterns through learning and experience. They develop problem-solving skills, social attachments, attitudes, preferences, and predispositions. There is even some evidence to suggest that they acquire a rudimentary form of abstract thinking. But according to conventional wisdom, apparently absent among other animals is the capacity for advanced forms of self-conceptualization (though not all scientists and animal caretakers agree on this point).

The self-concept in human beings is actually a composite of at least seven categories of perceptions. They consist of: (1) the *social* self, based on our interactions with others, (2) the *aspiring* self, something we are actively striving to become, (3) the *perfect* self, which we consider to be ideal but unattainable, (4) the *fluid* self, which we see as constantly changing, (5) the *actual* self, which we experience as our total self at the moment, (6) the *psychic* self, which we see as the composite of our multiple psychic faculties, and (7) the *higher* self, which we see as the product of our highest attributes and potentials.

The unique human capacity for perceiving and understanding the multiple facets of the self is an integral component of the psychic empowerment perspective. Our perceptions of the self affect the quality of our existence, with positive perceptions of the self always conducive to personal growth and well-being. Among the important goals of psychic empowerment are increased self-awareness and positive self-perceptions.

The Psychic Self-perception Procedure recognizes our intuitive capacity to experience the total self and each of its components, including the aura. The procedure is designed to activate those inner resources required to generate a valid representation of our own aura. It attempts to promote a deeper understanding of the personal aura and its relevance to the total self. Essentially meditative in nature, the procedure requires a willingness to explore the innermost self with honesty and objectivity. Here is the procedure:

Step 1. Preliminaries. Find a comfortable place, and set aside approximately thirty minutes for the procedure. Give yourself permission to relax and explore your innermost thoughts and feelings.

Step 2. Mental Passivity. Close your eyes and take in a few deep breaths, exhaling slowly. Extinguish all active thought.

Step 3. Inner Awareness. Focus your full attention on the center of energy within your deepest, innermost being. With your thoughts now turned inward, sense the energy emanating from the aura's inner core, permeating your total being and surrounding your physical body with a radiant glow.

Step 4. Aura Scan. Visualize your aura and mentally scan it, beginning with the energy patterns above your head and progressively working your way downward. Notice the sensations and impressions that accompany the aura scan.

Step 5. Aura Contemplation. Contemplate first upon the full aura, and then focus on specific areas and characteristics. Allow insight to spontaneously emerge either as impressions or images. Pay particular attention to the psychic knowledge that almost always emerges during this process.

Step 6. Internalization. Internalize the experience by taking a mental snapshot of your aura and file it away in your mind for future reference. Conclude the procedure with the affirmation: *I am fully empowered with positive energy.*

By simply retrieving the aura image generated and stored in memory by this procedure, you can instantly re-active the empowering effects of aura self-perception. Among the typical results are deeper insight into the self, a sense of well-being, and feelings of personal worth.

Awareness of the aura is sometimes reported by subjects during certain altered states of consciousness, including the out-of-body state and hypnosis. Out-of-body experiences (OBEs), also known as astral projection and astral travel, occur when the astral or non-biological body disengages its biological counterpart, and in that disengaged form, experiences distant spatial realities independent of the physical body. Subjects who enter the out-of-body state often report seeing their physical body at rest enveloped in a glow of energy. Our studies revealed, however, that the aura around the physical body during the out-of-body state is markedly different from the aura as seen during normal consciousness. Among the common alterations are changes in energy distribution and coloration. Since these alterations continue for the duration of the out-of-body experience, it would follow that the use of out-of-body procedures for viewing and interpreting one's own aura is of limited value. In contrast to OBEs, hypnosis as a typically receptive state presents a unique opportunity for viewing and intervening into the aura system. A later chapter is devoted to hypnosis and its relevance to the aura.

In summary, we can each develop our capacity to view the aura, whether that of another person or our own. Our success in interpreting the aura, and more importantly, intervening into its functions to achieve our empowerment goals, depends largely on our ability to see the aura. Only through practice and experience can we master that critical skill.

4

Interpreting the Aura

It is the glory of God to conceal a thing, but the glory
of kings is to search a thing out.

—Proverbs 25:2
(Amplified version)

THE HUMAN AURA, perhaps more than any other single human characteristic, signals the eminence of our existence as an immortal life force in the universe. It reflects the splendor of our origins and the magnificent master plan within which we all exist. The aura is, indeed, the stuff of life itself. Simply seeing the human aura and experiencing its beauty are empowering, but discovering the aura's full relevance requires a deeper look into of its essential features and complex processes.

Like the physical body, the human aura exists as a interactive system with many parts and functions. Even its most minute, obscure element can be important to the greater whole. A full interpretation of the aura must consider each component and its relevance to the total system.

Interpreting Color in the Aura

From a historical perspective, most ancient cultures used color as an important symbol or perceived source of power. Even their gods had certain colors as symbols of their deity and power. Many cultures believed that color had magical value, particularly in the art of healing. Also, the use of different colors to signify such traits as bravery, loyalty, status, and devotion was a widespread tradition.

Even today, colors are still used among the world's most advanced cultures to signify various social and religious concepts. Among the common examples are white to signify purity, green to signify life, red to signify courage, and black to signify grief. In colleges and universities, colors are used to indicate different branches of learning. In the military, various colors and color combinations have special meanings as signals and codes.

At a personal level, our emotions and sensations are strongly influenced by different colors. Certain colors are exciting, others are calming. Most of us find pleasure in some colors, and displeasure in others. Research has shown that certain colors have appetite appeal, whereas others appeal to the sense of smell. Still others are neutral in their appeal. Most people have a favorite color, with blue being the most highly preferred.

Perhaps not surprisingly, coloration is one of the most critical attributes of the human aura. Color in the aura provides a visible manifestation of energy, with each color variation designating a particular energy function. Although a dominant color, which can envelop the total body, is commonly observed in the aura, multiple colors spanning the visible color spectrum will occasionally appear. In the rainbow aura, various colors are arranged in spherical layers enveloping the body, with each layer having its own distinct borders, or else blending softly with other layers to produce border regions of mixed coloration. Colors in the aura can appear as disorganized blotches that fade into other colors, or they may form distinct bodies of isolated color. Although the human aura is never totally white or totally black, areas of white or black will occasionally appear somewhere in the aura. These colors are usually evident as concentrated points of light or darkness rather than extensive regions.

Aside from the distribution of color, the intensity, expansiveness, and clarity of colors in the aura will also vary widely. Occasionally, small concentrations of extremely brilliant, iridescent color will be noted in an otherwise unremarkable aura. Typically, the intensity and expansiveness of the color is a reliable index into the forcefulness of its energy, with the more intense and expansive the color the stronger its influence and symbolic significance. The clarity or brightness of color is a useful index into the empowerment nature of the color, with the clearer or brighter the color the more empowering its influence on the person. Dullness or discoloration in the aura almost always signifies a disempowering or enfeebling influence.

In this chapter, we will explore the significance of various colors in the aura, with special focus on the relationship between coloration and personal traits. The conclusions presented here are based on careful, controlled viewings of the aura and comparisons of the observed coloration with other assessment results, including the subject's self-ratings as well as standardized evaluations, such as intelligence and personality testing.

In our studies of the aura, coloration was determined by a team of trained aura specialists who arrived at a consensus following a series of aura viewings for each experimental subject under carefully controlled conditions. Although our studies identified only a total of ten color categories, it is important to note that the potential for color variation in the aura is literally inexhaustible. It's possible that many colors and color arrangements will not be included in the following discussion.

The Rainbow

Any of the colors of the artists' palette can be represented in the rainbow aura. The rainbow pattern consists of a variety of colors arranged, often in tones of softness, to form a symmetrical rainbow enveloping either the full body or a particular body region, such as the head and shoulders. Typically bright and expansive, the rainbow aura suggests a diverse combination of many positive personal traits—intelligence, humanitarian concerns, social interests, intuitive knowledge, integrity, generosity, optimism, and self-actualization.

The person whose full aura is a highly brilliant rainbow of color tends to possess the best of all worlds. As a group, they are usually intensely committed and successful in their careers and personal lives. Many great leaders and social reformers of today have rainbow auras. As we will see later, new evidence based on retrospective strategies using numerology suggests that some of the most important historical figures of the past, including William Shakespeare and George Washington, also had rainbow auras.

While the rainbow aura usually signifies a myriad of highly desirable personal characteristics, it is exceptionally sensitive to imbalance and discoloration. Dinginess, while enfeebling to auras of any color pattern, is particularly detrimental to the rainbow aura. Also, the rainbow aura is especially vulnerable to abrupt interjections of new color, particularly red, that can temporarily disrupt the symmetry of its patterns.

Yellow

Yellow is one of the colors most commonly found in the human aura. It is often seen in abundance in the auras of individuals who are highly intelligent, sociable, and dependable. The brightness of the yellow is typically associated with intelligence, whereas the expansiveness of the color is typically associated with social competence and dependability. As a general rule, the brighter the color, the higher the intelligence, and the more expansive the color, the stronger the social skills.

In the predominantly yellow aura, the location of brilliance provides a useful index into the exact nature of the subject's intellectual make-up. Bright yellow around the head is associated with abstract thinking, problem solving, and verbal skills, whereas bright yellow around the shoulders and chest is associated with superior eye-hand coordination and mechanical skills.

As an index to interpersonal skills and social interests, the highly expansive yellow aura is almost always accompanied by such traits as dependability, friendliness, and empathy for others. Highly sociable individuals will almost invariably show an expansive glow of light yellow in the outermost region of the aura.

A combination of high intelligence and strong social skills is reflected in the aura by a bright inner region of rich yellow and an expansive outer region of light yellow. This pattern is often observed in the auras of powerful leaders and social activists. The combination of these color characteristics seems to empower them with the ideal blend of intellectual insight and social warmth required to influence people and bring forth change. They are especially skilled at sizing up situations and anticipating consequences. Our studies of political candidates found that campaign success could be predicted with a high degree of accuracy through simple analysis of coloration patterns in the candidate's aura.

Dullness and constriction in the predominantly yellow aura usually indicate highly stressful conditions that assert a negative influence on intellectual functions and social interactions. Thwarted academic or social strivings, excessive pressure to succeed, loss of social status, and interpersonal conflict invariably contract the aura and reduce its brightness. With the resolution of these issues, the aura typically regains its characteristic brilliance and expansiveness.

Blue

Another color commonly found in the human aura is blue. Shade and clarity are critical factors that determine the relevance of this important color. Light blue is associated with balance, tranquillity, flexibility, and optimism, whereas deep blue is associated with mental alertness and emotional control. Light blue in the aura is almost always found among subjects who value self-insight and empathy for others. The deeper shades of blue are often found in the auras of individuals who are sharp-witted and self-disciplined.

Blue coloration in the aura is particularly responsive to meditation and relaxation strategies that seem to literally generate bright energy and disperse it into the aura system. Strategies that include peaceful images of a clear blue sky are especially effective in producing light blue in the aura with an accompanying serene mood state. Strategies that include images of a deep blue pool have been developed to literally introduce deep blue into the aura while enhancing emotional stability and control. In the laboratory setting, biofeedback technology can objectively monitor the physiological changes, including alterations in brain wave patterns, that accompany these color changes in the aura.

Dull blue anywhere in the aura is associated with negative stress, pessimism, despondency, and insecurity. Deeply depressed and suicidal individuals will invariably have expansive areas of dark, dingy blue in their auras. The common expression, feeling blue, could have its origin in subconscious awareness of dull blue in the aura. Speculatively at least, a depressed mood state could literally generate dull blue energy and disperse it into the aura. Dull blue energy, once introduced into the aura, could in turn generate a more deeply depressed mood state. The result is a vicious cycle of chronic depression. Whatever the dynamics of the phenomenon, the relationship between aura color and mood state has important therapeutic implications for preventing and breaking the cycle of depression. In the next chapter, we will discuss empowerment strategies designed specifically to alleviate dullness and introduce brightness into the aura system.

Green

Bright green in the aura signifies healing energy, self-actualization strivings, and raised consciousness, particularly concerning global conditions. Typically, the auras of health care professionals—physicians, nurses, clinical and counseling psychologists, psychiatrists, psychic healers, and social workers—are predominantly bright green, or they will, at least, include large areas of bright green. Interestingly, the auras of psychic healers are usually iridescent, a feature not always found in the auras of other health care specialists. Bright iridescent green is also associated with the magickal dimensions of consciousness, and is usually found in abundance in the auras of practitioners of magick.

As might be expected, bright green is commonly found in the auras of students planning careers in the health care fields. In our studies of medical students, bright green was the most frequently observed aura color, although other colors were usually present. Also, in a study of students enrolled in a nursing program, bright green in the aura was observed with greater frequency than any other color.

Environmentalists tend to have expansive regions of bright green in their auras. Among highly committed environmental activists, bright green will often appear as a sphere of radiant energy enveloping the full body.

Dull green in the human aura is related to pessimism, inner conflict, and personal unfulfillment. Dull green is also the color of envy, thus suggesting a basis for the common expression, "green with envy." Individuals with large regions of dull green in their auras tend to complain of injustice and the unfairness of people around them. They are quick to rationalize their behavior and blame others for their failures, but they are seldom overtly hostile. In fact, the negative impulses signified by this color are often suppressed or buried in the subconscious. In many cases, the animosity they feel toward others appears to be a displacement of their negative feelings toward themselves. Perhaps not surprisingly, individuals whose auras are predominantly dull green tend to resist change while rejecting the negative implications of this color.

A very dull green with shades of gray discoloration is often a precursor of personal catastrophe or other serious adversity, including physical illness.

Pink

Pink is the color of youth, rejuvenation, sensitivity, idealism, and talent. Although it may appear among other colors that are dull or discolored, pink in the aura is always bright and radiant. It is a hopeful color, and it tends to be relatively stable. Its correlates include a positive outlook on life, versatility, and a strong self-image.

Because it is found with great frequency in the auras of centenarians, pink is often associated with longevity. Among the most effective rejuvenating strategies for both men and women are those expressly designed to add pink to the aura.

Pink is often found in abundance in the auras of men and women with expressed humanitarian interests. Typically, they have achieved prominence in their careers, and they are usually generous in contributing their time and resources to causes they consider worthwhile. They are usually moderate in their political views, and they tend to focus their interests on activities such as historical preservation and the arts.

Brown

Brown in the human aura is associated with a strong interest in the earth and its natural resources along with such personality traits as practicality, stability, and independence. Geologists, ecologists, archaeologists, landscapers, and construction workers almost always have regions of brown in their auras, which can appear as either an isolated area or an enveloping sphere among other colors.

Individuals with considerable brown in the aura are usually interested in outdoor activities such as hiking, skiing, mountain climbing, and hunting. They are often successful Generation Xers, but they are prone to express dissatisfaction with the routine activities of their careers and life in the suburbs. They are usually health conscious. Working out in the gym and racquetball are among their common after-hours activities. On weekends, they often escape to the beach or a mountain retreat. Although they are usually sociable and friendly, they value privacy and space.

The successful entrepreneur and self-made millionaire will invariably have auras with significant areas of brown. CEOs with this color are usually assertive, practical, and independent. They believe in themselves and they rely heavily on their intuitive skills. Although they surround themselves with highly talented subordinates and advisers, they are self-assured, decisive, and competent decision-makers. While they are not impulsive, they are skilled at "striking while the iron is hot."

As a cautionary note, brown in the aura should not be confused with the discoloration associated with cigarette smoking. As previously mentioned, cigarette smoke, whether inhaled or externally absorbed, constricts the aura and discolors it with an overlay of dingy, yellowish brown.

Purple

Purple, a relatively rare color in the aura, is associated with philosophical and abstract interests. Persons with this aura coloration are often creative and artistic. They value intuitive knowledge above the opinions of experts who, they note, often disagree among themselves. They are usually generalists who focus on broad principles rather than specific facts or claims based on statistical data which they tend to distrust.

Although they usually consider material assets to be of secondary importance, wealth seems to come easily to them. They are typically above average in intelligence, and they possess superior verbal skills. They almost always command respect from their peers, and they usually settle into comfortable careers in which they are free to pursue their personal interests.

Purple is often predominant in the auras of ministers, philosophers, and theoreticians. It is a highly stable color that tends to resist discoloration.

Orange

The predominantly orange aura is usually found among people who are strong achievers. They are usually social extroverts who tend to pursue careers that require considerable social interaction, such as in politics and sales. They are usually independent and competitive, and they almost always possess strong persuasive skills. They tend to overcompensate for their felt weaknesses, and they may become defensive when faced with criticism. Although they value positive social interactions, they often experience difficulty establishing long-term relationships. Their energies are sometimes scattered, and they often fail to complete important tasks.

Discoloration in the orange aura is associated with impatience, egotism, a low tolerance for frustration, and emotional instability.

Gray

Gray in the aura is a typically transient but foreboding color. It can foreshadow illness, adversity, and when expansive throughout the aura, even death. Impending illness is usually indicated by grayish discoloration in the innermost region of the aura. Small areas of dark gray can signify a particularly serious health problems, such as an organ dysfunction, depending on the location of the color.

Gray can also signal non-health related adversity, particularly when it appears in the upper region of a constricted aura. An expansive outer region of gray is often associated with personal loss involving either finances or relationships.

Red

Red in the aura occurs typically as either a sudden flash or a relatively small but intense area of transient coloration. It is often associated with impulsive behavior and strong emotion, including outbursts of anger. Like feeling blue and green with envy, the common expression "seeing red" to signify anger may have a literal basis in the aura. Highly intense flashes of red in the aura as signals of anger could command our attention, either consciously or subconsciously, thus resulting in a mental association.

Although flashes of red in the aura are usually transient, strands of red can become woven into the aura as relatively permanent patterns of activity with potentially disempowering consequences. In our studies of prison inmates, streaks of red appeared frequently in the auras of men who were repeat offenders or who had been convicted of violent crimes. Streaks of red were also noted frequently in the auras of adolescents who tended to act out their aggressive impulses.

In our studies of college students, a significant relationship was found between areas of red in the aura and the need for excitement and adventure as measured by psychological tests. Areas of red were also associated with restlessness and risk-taking behavior. Although areas of red were found infrequently in the auras of college students in general, they were not uncommon in the auras of male students who were highly active in contact sports.

Color and Numerology

Any relationship between numerology, or the science of numbers, and the human aura might seem at first suspect. But if the world is built on the power of numbers, as claimed by Pythagoras in 550 b.c., and if each number possesses significance beyond its expression of quantity, as claimed by Agrippa two thousand years later, it should not be surprising to find that the energy frequencies of numbers could, in some ways, relate to the energy frequencies of the aura. Such relationships have, in fact, been found.

In a study conducted in our laboratory, the birthdate for each of fifty subjects was reduced to a single digit using a modified numerological procedure, which we will later illustrate. The predominant color of the aura was then determined for each subject by a panel of trained aura viewers. Comparisons between the aura's predominant color and the subject's birth number revealed a very powerful relationship, with the birth number providing a useful index into the aura's predominant color. Further comparisons revealed a strong agreement between the birth number's numerological meaning and the significance of predominant color in the aura. Stated another way, the personal traits associated with a given individual's birth number were similar to the personal traits associated with that individual's predominant aura color. Two replications of the study revealed similar relationships. As a result of these studies, if given only an individual's birth number, we can predict with reasonable confidence the predominant color of that individual's aura.

Following is a summary of our findings concerning the relationship between birth number and color in the aura.

Birth Number 1. Individuals with a birth number of 1 were typically found to have a predominantly orange aura. Both the number 1 and the color orange signify independence and a strong achievement drive.

Birth Number 2. A birth number of 2 was found with great frequency among individual's whose auras were predominantly light blue. Both the number 2 and light blue in the aura signify balance and tranquillity.

Birth Number 3. Pink and the birth number 3 were often found together, both of which signify talent and versatility.

Birth Number 4. A predominantly brown aura was found for individuals who had a birth number of 4. Both the brown aura and the birth number 4 signify steadiness and practicality.

Birth Number 5. The rainbow aura is associated with the birth number 5. Although red was found from time to time in most of the auras we studied, it was observed with slightly greater frequency in the auras of individuals who had a birth number of 5. Both the rainbow aura with its occasional red pattern and the number five are associated with diversity, intensity, and excitement.

Birth Number 6. The predominantly yellow aura was found frequently among individuals with a birth number of 6, both of which signify dependability, intelligence, and social competence.

Birth Number 7. The birth number 7 was associated with the predominantly purple aura, both of which are associated with abstract interests.

Birth Number 8. The birth number 8, which signifies success, was found with great frequency for individuals whose auras combined green and yellow. The constellation of traits associated with green and yellow, like the number 8, suggests a strong potential for success.

Birth Number 9. Green and the birth number 9 were often found together, both of which suggest self-actualization strivings and global concerns.

When taken together, our studies of the relationship between numerology and the human aura suggest that one's birth number represents broad categories of growth resources and potentials, whereas the make-up of the personal aura signifies the specific nature of one's capacities and achievements, with coloration in the aura monitoring the growth process. The characteristics associated with a given birth number exist on a growth continuum, with the related coloration in the aura reflecting the developmental level of those characteristics. A low developmental level, even when potentials are high, is typically reflected by either an absence of brilliance in the aura or constriction in the aura pattern. When the positive aspects of characteristics associated with a given birth number are fully developed, the aura's color related to that birth number assumes an expansive and rare brilliance that many aura viewers describe as prismatic. At the lower end of the continuum, the color related to a particular birth number becomes diluted and characteristically deficient in brilliance. Nevertheless, the growth possibilities suggested by both the color and birth number remain intact.

For our studies, determining the birth number required assigning a single digit value to each individual's date of birth. Our preliminary studies found that neither the birth number based on the birth month's position in the year nor the exact color/number relationship commonly held by numerology was significantly related to the dominant aura color as observed by our team of specialists. As a result, we used procedures that departed somewhat from traditional numerology.

To determine birth number, our adaptation applied certain aspects of numerology commonly used to determine an individual's name number. A numerical value was first assigned to each letter in the month of birth, depending on the letter's position in the alphabet, rather than assigning a numerical value to the month based on the month's position in the year. For letters with two digit numbers, the digits were added together until they were reduced to a single digit which was then assigned to the letter. For instance, the letter V occupies the 13th position in the alphabet. When the number 13 is reduced to a single digit, the letter V assumes a numerical value of 4. Letters occupying a single digit position automatically assume the numerical value of that position. The letter G, for instance, occupies the 7th position in the alphabet and thus automatically assumes a single digit numerical value of 7. The following number/alphabet key commonly used in numerology provides a quick reference to each letter's automatic or reduced single digit value.

```
A B C D E F G H I
J K L M N O P Q R
S T U V W X Y Z -
1 2 3 4 5 6 7 8 9
```

As can be seen from this key, the letters A, J, and S have a numerical value of l; the letters B, K, and T, have a numerical value of 2; and so forth. To arrive at a total numerical value for the date of birth, the numerical values of all letters in the month of birth are added to the numbers in the day and year of birth. The numbers in that total value are than added together until the sum is reduced to a single digit. For a birth date of September 16, 1975, the single digit birth date number is computed as follows:

S E P T E M B E R 1 6 1 9 7 5 =
$1+5+7+2+5+4+2+5+9+1+6+1+9+7+5 = 69 = 6+9 = 15 = 1+5 = 6$

Using this formula, the individual in our example has a birth number of 6.

In our study, the birth number for each subject was compared to the dominant color in the subject's aura. Finally, the numerological significance of the number was compared to the auraological significance of the predominant aura color in order to determine the level of agreement between these two indicators. For our demonstration subject, the aura turned out to be predominantly yellow. Since the birth number 6 and the yellow aura both signify social and intellectual competence, the two measures were found to be in agreement. Tending to validate that finding was the fact that our subject was an honor student. We therefore found agreement among three important variables—birth number, predominant aura color, and personal trait as signified by both.

As already noted, our studies of numerology and the aura suggest that an individual's birth number alone (as determined by our adapted procedure) provides a useful and convenient index into the predominant aura color, including that of individuals who are unavailable for viewing. Even the aura coloration of important historical figures could be predicted with reasonably accuracy using this procedure as a retrospective strategy, provided we had the individual's date of birth. The table that follows presents the predicted dominant aura colors for selected historical figures.

Historical Figure	Date of Birth	Birth Number	Aura Color
Washington, George	February 22, 1732	5	Rainbow
Lincoln, Abraham	February 12, 1809	9	Green
Elizabeth II	April 21, 1926	5	Rainbow
Bell, Alexander G.	March 3, 1847	3	Pink
Dickens, Charles	February 7, 1812	7	Purple
Einstein, Albert	March 14, 1879	9	Green
Kennedy, John F.	May 9, 1917	3	Pink
Shakespeare, William	April 23(?), 1564	5	Rainbow
Freud, Sigmund	May 6, 1856	2	Blue
Franklin, Benjamin	January 17, 1706	4	Brown
Hawthorne, Nathaniel	July 4, 1804	5	Rainbow
Hemingway, Ernest	July 21, 1899	9	Green

Aside from its usefulness in assigning dominant aura colors to persons not physically present, numerology is important in our study of the human aura because it supplements other strategies, including direct aura viewing techniques. There is no one best way to study the human aura. Given a repertoire of strategies, we can compensate for the weaknesses that are often inherent in a given approach. Also, optional strategies can be useful in validating the accuracy of other procedures. For instance, if given the birth number of the individual whose aura we are viewing, we could infer the subject's predominant aura color, thereby helping us test the accuracy our aura viewing strategies. Of equal importance, we can use numerology as a supplement to our self-viewing efforts.

It is important to emphasize that the relationship between birth numbers and the aura colors associated with them is of limited usefulness except when interpreted within the context of the total aura system and other sources of information available to us. Because the studies relating numerology to the human aura are limited, and since the relationships are not perfect, our conclusions must be considered tentative at best. Further research is needed to increase our understanding of this interesting phenomenon.

We have discussed only a few of the colors found in the human aura. Coloration in the aura is a dynamic function rather than simply a set of limited categories. The human eye can see a million or more different colors, each of which can be present in the human aura, and each of which can possess empowerment relevance. We have focused on the significance of a limited number of selected colors in an effort, not to exhaust all the possibilities, but rather to provide a general foundation upon which we can expand our awareness and understanding of the aura.

The Aura Signature

Aside from color, the human aura consists of numerous other critical elements which, when properly interpreted, can increase our understanding of the aura and its relevance to our personal empowerment. Each aura feature, including those laden with potential, is responsive to our intervention. Perhaps more than any other human system, the aura holds the master key that can open the door to a deeper understanding of the innermost part of our being and the outermost reaches of the universe, while at once connecting us to both.

Simply becoming aware of the aura and its functions inspires us with a new appreciation of the magnificent life force within us. But by probing each of the aura's essential features and exploring its empowering relevance, we discover new and exciting possibilities for our personal growth and fulfillment.

Energy Patterns and Designs

Energy, which can be defined simply as an effective force, is the essence of the human aura system. Rather than a single energy phenomenon, the human aura is a constellation of many energy components and processes. The energies of the aura are typically visible during viewing as a colorful glow that then assumes highly structured patterns and designs of energy activity. Together, these elements form a unique structure called the aura signature for each individual. Although the aura is constantly evolving and changing, the aura signature, like personality, is relatively stable.

The aura is influenced by many complex interactions, both within the aura system itself and between the aura and other influences. The aura signature provides a useful index into the nature of those interactions. Symmetry in the signature, for instance, suggests mental, physical, and spiritual harmony, while turbulence in the signature suggests an agitated, unbalanced state.

Any viewing strategy that reveals such aura characteristics as coloration and magnitude is usually effective in uncovering the full make-up of the aura. Occasionally, highly specific structural components will become visible during aura viewing, even before the emergence of color and other more general features. Among the commonly observed signature designs and patterns found in the aura are the following: (1) *streams of energy*, (2) *clusters of energy*, (3) *points of light*, (4) *points of darkness*, (5) *voids*, (6) *agitation*, (7) *symmetry* and *balance*, (8) *fissures*, (9) *tentacles*, (10) *arcs*, and (11) a wide range of *unique energy formations*, including a variety of geometric bodies of energy.

The notion of an intricate aura system with complex signature patterns and designs may, at first, seem somewhat farfetched, but when we consider the intricate complexity of the biological body, we are not surprised to find equal complexity in the human aura system. Also, when we scan the universe, form the largest known galaxy to the smallest particle of matter, we find a magnificent system that is comparable in many ways to the wondrous design of our own being, including the make-up of our aura system. Like the cosmos, we are a complex creation of many elements, all designed to function in harmony.

Interpreting the signature design of the aura requires not only skill in viewing the aura, but an acute awareness of specific elements and their interactions. In the following discussion, we will explore several major aura signature characteristics and their importance to our personal empowerment. Many of our conclusions are based on laboratory investigations which included direct viewings, psychological testing, and interviews. For our studies, the volunteer subjects, all college students, were first administered a battery of psychological tests. Aura viewings were then conducted by a panel of trained aura specialists. Upon arriving at a consensus regarding the aura's signature characteristics for each participant, the viewers conducted interviews with the subject to gather additional information, and then compared the specific characteristics of the aura with the interview and psychological test results.

Streams of Energy

Glowing streams, which are commonly believed to distribute energy, can occur in a variety of formations and colors anywhere in the aura. They can radiate outward as brilliant, symmetrical streamers from the aura's inner regions, or they can meander throughout the aura in a network of gleaming veins of energy. Broad streams of sparkling energy often follow the borders of various color regions. For instance, if the aura includes a region of blue enveloping the full body with an outer region of green, distinct border streams of bright energy will often characterize the merging of the two color regions. Occasionally, smaller energy streams are visible as isolated currents of activity which can occur anywhere in the aura. Small but intensely bright streams are often observed around the subject's head and shoulders.

Energy streams, which are usually tingling to the touch when active, can become blocked, thus restricting the aura's energizing capacity. The result is a loss of energy, inefficiency, and in instances of prolonged blockage, even physical illness. Our studies found that individuals with blockages in the aura system almost always experience chronic fatigue, difficulty concentrating, and irritability. They often complain of exhaustion and inability to complete routine daily tasks.

Blockages are visible in the aura as interruptions or barriers in the stream's continuous flow of energy. A blocked stream is typically characterized by dullness which replaces the characteristic brightness of the stream's energy. The aura massage, discussed in a later chapter, can effectively unleash blocked energy in the aura, while alleviating the symptoms associated with the blockage.

Clusters of Energy

Clusters are relatively intense concentrations of colorful energy which, like streams, can occur anywhere in the aura. They are often seen as bright, intermeshing symmetrical networks of energy that assemble in the aura's outer regions. To the touch, as during the aura massage, they are typically warm and vibrant.

Although they can become permanent fixtures in the aura, clusters typically enter the aura system temporarily, apparently to meet highly specific empowerment needs. The color and location of the cluster can be a clue to its significance. Our studies of college students revealed frequent glowing clusters of yellow energy near the head region, a location that suggested a cognitive empowerment role. In instances of injury or physical illness, a bright green cluster will often appear spontaneously at the site of impairment, illustrated by an athlete who had recently sustained an injury to the Achilles tendon. An iridescent green cluster, which appeared to radiate healing energy, was clearly visible in his aura at the area of injury.

Bright clusters are at times thought to be cosmic injections of power into the aura system. When they appear in the external region of our energy field, they are believed to have preparatory significance, often energizing us for a future challenge or new venture. For instance, a candidate for public office developed an unusually large cluster of bright orange energy in his outer aura, a pattern that apparently energized his remarkably successful campaign.

A bright cluster of blue energy is often found in the inner aura region of persons who are facing adversity, such as the break-up of a relationship or loss of a loved one. Whatever the nature of the demands, the aura seems to rise to the occasion. The empowered aura gathers the essential resources, whether from within the self or from higher cosmic sources, and organizes them to meet our energy needs. We will later discuss ways of bringing totally new clusters of aura power into our lives.

Points of Light

Points of light in the aura are usually associated with powerful forces that intervene to empower our lives. According to some experienced aura viewers, a point of light in the aura can signify the presence of a spiritual influence, such as a ministering guide or guardian angel. That possibility was illustrated by a student whose aura revealed a bright point of light over his shoulder soon after he narrowly escaped serious injury in an auto accident. He interpreted the point of light as a clear manifestation of his guardian angel. Bright points of light can also be seen as concentrated energy fragments dispersed by the aura's inner core of pure energy. As spin-off fragments, they are believed to be spontaneously projected into the aura to meet emergency needs or unexpected energy demands, such as a personal crisis or sudden illness.

Although small in size, points of bright light usually command our attention when we view the aura. While they can occur anywhere in the aura, they are observed with greater frequency in the aura's upper region or at the center of an energy cluster. Occasionally the point is seen directly over the head, a placement which is thought to signify self-actualization strivings or spiritual enlightenment. When they appear elsewhere in the aura, the point is believed to signify an important influence or achievement—past, present, or future.

In our past-life regression studies, subjects with isolated points of light in their auras often discovered important past-life experiences that they related to the points. In a very interesting case, the regression subject whose aura had a point of light in the chest region discovered that in a past life, she had been stabbed and mortally wounded in the chest while protecting her lover. To her, the point of light shining out from the darkness of her past represented, not tragedy, but a protective presence in her current life.

Points of Darkness

Occasionally, a point of darkness will appear in the aura. While points of light suggest positive influences, including the infusion of positive energy into the aura, points of darkness suggest either a negative attack on the aura or a severe weakness in the aura system. Points of darkness in the aura often appear as puncture wounds that signal psychic trauma or the recent invasion of a negative force. As we will see later, some underdeveloped aura systems are known to tap into other aura systems, thereby draining the host victim of energy and leaving behind a temporary dark point in the aura. Dark points associated with this phenomenon, sometimes called psychic vampirism, are usually surrounded by a grayish discoloration that indicates a serious depletion of aura energy. In a later chapter, we will explore psychic vampirism in greater depth.

A dark point in the aura is also associated with a particular vulnerability or deficiency. In contrast to puncture wounds, the surrounding aura under this condition typically shows no discoloration. The dark point in this context is the aura's equivalent of an Achilles' heel—its enfeebling effects are characteristically limited, but with potential for larger consequences. Common examples are inferiority complexes, phobias, and addictions.

Voids

Voids, which are more expansive than points, are non-functional, inactive areas in the aura with little or no energy supply or capacity to generate new energy. They can occur anywhere in the aura, typically as colorless, transparent regions with no indication of aura activity. When they occur in the aura's outer regions, they suggest vulnerability to external threats. When they appear in the aura's inner zones, they are often associated with feelings of emptiness. They can represent unfulfilled strivings, discouragement, and loss of hope. Extensive voids are often found in the aura of people who experience identity diffusion, depersonalization, and detachment from others.

Although voids can be transient, they tend to be relatively permanent unless positive action is taken to uncover the source of the void and activate the aura's capacity for renewal and completeness. As we will find in a later chapter, aura strategies have been developed to expand the elasticity of the aura and specifically empower it to bridge voids, thereby restoring the aura's full capacities. These strategies, which usually include appropriate affirmations, are effective in not only closing voids but also resolving the underlying issues related to them.

Agitation

As a highly sensitive energy system, the human aura is often vulnerable to agitating influences that can disrupt its functions. Like many other aura characteristics, agitation in the aura's energy patterns can originate from within the self or from external sources. These energy disturbances can occur throughout the aura system, or they can be limited to an isolated area of the aura. Whether localized or general in nature, they are usually visible to the experienced viewer as a churning turbulence accompanied by dull discoloration. Fractured relationships, insecurity, fear, and excessive anxiety are examples of influences that can agitate the aura.

Our studies of college students found that unresolved conflict accompanied by guilt is particularly disruptive to the aura. This was illustrated by a student who felt responsible for the death of his fiancée in an auto crash. For many months following the tragedy, his aura reflected the turbulence of his grief and guilt.

Localized disruptions in the aura are sometimes associated with physical disorders, with the location of the turbulence often signaling the nature of the disorder. Chronic pain is almost always reflected in the aura as a localized disruption of energy at the site of pain. For instance, an engineer who experienced chronic pain from a knee injury showed agitation accompanied by discoloration in his aura at the location of the pain. While the localized agitation in the aura was always present, it dramatically increased during episodes of severe pain. In another instance, a teacher who complained of stomach problems showed abdominal agitation in her aura. We will later discuss strategies that reduce agitation and use the energies of the aura to manage both mental and physical pain.

In some instances, an apparent agitated pattern in the aura is a positive response to the demands of an urgent situation. In that context, what appears to be a disturbance in the aura is, in reality, a constructive mobilization of aura energy. In a remarkable instance of this phenomenon, a champion chess player immediately prior to competition showed extensive activity in the uppermost region of his aura, a reflection of the cognitive vigilance and energy mobilization demanded by the upcoming event. The stirred-up state seen during constructive mobilization, unlike other forms of agitation, is typically accompanied by brightness instead of dull discoloration in the aura.

Symmetry

Symmetry emanates from the aura's inner core to permeate the aura with bright, flowing energy that is evenly distributed throughout the aura system. Typically absent in the symmetrical aura are voids, fissures, and agitation, each of which can disrupt the positive flow of energy.

Symmetry in the human aura signals a healthy, harmonious mind, body, and spirit interaction. As we move toward harmony within ourselves, the aura system responds by shifting toward symmetry and balance. The result is an empowerment cycle in which the symmetrical aura enriches our lives with greater power and new possibilities for personal fulfillment.

The symmetrical aura system is flexible and responsive to change. As the convergence of mental, physical, and spiritual energy, the symmetrical aura is a powerhouse of adaptation and growth. The full actualization of our potentials depends largely on our capacity to accommodate change and internalize new learning experiences. A symmetrical, balanced aura system facilitates that critical process.

Our investigations of symmetry in the aura revealed a two-way interaction between learning and symmetry, with each contributing to the other. We found that the auras of college students enrolled in freshmen remedial programs became increasingly bright and symmetrical as they acquired the skills considered essential to academic success at the college level. This phenomenon was particular evident among students enrolled in a special Summer Start Program at Athens State College (now Athens State University). The highly successful program, which was specifically structured to prepare non-admissible applicants for admission to the regular college program, included meditation activities designed to promote a state of symmetry and balance.

Given the interaction between symmetry and learning, it requires no quantum leap to conclude that aura intervention strategies designed to induce symmetry in the aura could directly accelerate learning. Strategies have, in fact, been developed specifically to achieve that goal. In the next chapter, we will discuss the Cosmic Centering Procedure which has been successfully applied in a variety of educational settings to accelerate cognitive growth and promote scholastic achievement.

Fissures

Fissures, including breaks and tears, typically originate in the outer areas of the aura. Unlike voids, fissures have jagged, irregular edges, and they are usually gray in coloration. Typically wedge-shaped, they can extend to the aura's innermost regions. Only rarely will the fissure originate in the aura's inner region. Fissures of inner origin are usually accompanied by dull discoloration not only within the fissure but throughout the aura.

Fissures in the aura are almost always the result of psychic injury that literally altered the aura's basic structure. They are often associated with trauma related to either early childhood or past-life experiences. Fissures are found frequently in the auras of men and women who, as children, were emotionally or physically abused, and they are common in the auras of battered women. Fissures in the aura are also associated with betrayal by a significant other, including a trusted friend or lover.

Many fissures are relatively permanent and resist efforts to correct them. To be effective, strategies designed to close the fissure must focus on underlying causes and the effects of the fissure on the total aura system, including the central energy core. Techniques focusing only on the fissure as a symptom can be effective in helping the subject to feel better, but unless underlying causes and their effects are considered, the results are temporary.

When the fissure is past-life related, hypnotic regression can be effective in uncovering the origin of the fissure and resolving the past-life issues related to it. The effects of past-life experiences survive, and they are reflected in the aura, sometimes as serious flaws. For instance, a law student with a large fissure of inner origin in his aura discovered during past-life regression that he had actively participated in the Spanish Inquisition as a tribunal judge who vigorously supported the Inquisition's activities. Given new insight through regression, he successfully worked through the negative residue of his past-life experiences. Almost immediately, the fissure in his aura began to diminish, and eventually, it vanished altogether. He partly attributes his current interest in law to a pressing need to counterbalance the injustices of his past-life actions.

Tentacles

Occasionally, tentacles extending outward from the aura's normal external boundaries will be observed in the human aura. They are often associated with immaturity and dependency needs. When they occur in the discolored aura, they are usually seen as either a plea for help or a need for support. Tentacles are frequently found in the auras of individuals who thrive on immediate gratification, or who make selfish and unreasonable demands on others.

Tentacles are often noted in the auras of pseudo-intellectuals who are egocentric and deficient in self-insight. These self-anointed "scholars" have neglected their own development, and they are usually critical of the achievements of others. They thrive on publicity and recognition, particularly as "expert debunkers" of psychic knowledge, yet they usually lack sufficient information to mount a convincing argument. They promote themselves as "skeptical thinkers," but they are typically rigid in their views, cynical of gifted psychics, and intolerant of persons whose thinking differs from their own. They tend to manipulate others, often shading the truth or stooping to deception to achieve their goals. They resist change, and they usually have serious difficulty establishing positive, long-term relationships.

The tentacled aura is often associated with psychic vampirism in which the deficient aura locks into the aura system of others who are in close proximity. This phenomenon is usually spontaneous, but it can be deliberate. Either way, it literally drains the host aura, depleting it of critical energy. The result for the psychic vampire is an instant energy surge; the unfortunate result for the victim is fatigue, and in instances of prolonged depletion, illness unless corrective action is taken. As previously noted, points of darkness in the aura can signal a recent psychic vampire attack that sucked energy from the aura. In a later chapter, we will develop strategies for counteracting psychic vampirism.

Arcs

An arc of bright energy is sometimes seen connecting two aura systems, a phenomenon that suggest a positive and potentially empowering interaction. Unlike tentacles that invade another aura system, arcs are positive expressions of warmth and compatibility. Any exchange of energy accompanying this phenomenon is always mutually empowering.

Typically seen connecting the upper regions of two aura systems, the arc is associated with close and satisfying social interactions. As a social phenomenon, the arc signals a mutually rewarding two-way relationship of giving and receiving. It is usually a transient phenomenon that occurs only intermittently during positive social interactions.

The arc is often seen between couples whose energy systems are congruous and whose relationship is fulfilling. It is important to note, however, that the absence of the arc does not signal the lack of positive interaction. When the spatial distance between two persons is slight, the arc can be replaced by a literal merging of the two aura systems. As expected, two auras that repel each other usually generate spatial distance between the systems and do not arc.

The arc will sometimes connect two outside regions within a given subject's own aura system. Under that condition, the arc is either protecting an area of vulnerability in the aura, or it is attempting to balance the aura's energy distribution. When a void appears in the aura's outer region, the arc is often seen spanning the void's external edges, as if attempting to repair the aura by closing the void.

Other Energy Patterns

A wide range of other energy patterns, including various geometric forms of energy, are often seen in the human aura. Typically intense in coloration and brightness, geometric energy forms can occur anywhere in the aura's energy field. These forms are thought to be either energy subfields or specialized concentrations of energy which can originate from either within the subject or an external source.

Spheres of energy are among the most common geometric forms found in the aura. Like other aura signature forms, the color and location of the sphere can offer clues to its energizing role. For instance, a bright yellow sphere of energy in the upper region of the aura is usually associated with intellectual enrichment. As we will see in a later chapter, structured intervention strategies focusing on intellectual development often introduce a glowing sphere of yellow energy into the aura's upper region. Our studies of college students found that aura intervention strategies which introduced a bright yellow sphere into the upper aura literally increased intelligence as measured by standardized tests.

A bright green sphere of energy in the aura is believed to generate healing energy, with the location of the sphere typically indicating the physical region being energized. Pre- and post-viewings of subjects who underwent psychic healing often reveal the introduction of an iridescent sphere of green energy in the affected body region. Many reputable psychic healers report that they deliberately generate a sphere of green healing energy which they, in turn, transfer to the recipient. We will later discuss strategies specifically designed to introduce healing energy into the aura.

Another energy form often found in the aura is the pyramid. Gifted psychics frequently have a bright pyramid of energy somewhere in the upper region of the aura, often directly overhead. Many psychic healers believe that they draw directly from a pyramid-like concentration of aura energy which they then transfer to the subject as healing energy. Our studies found that the geometric designs formed by lines in an individual's palm will often appear somewhere in the aura. Not unexpectedly, the pyramid or triangle pattern is almost always found in the palms of gifted psychics.

Not all geometric energy patterns found in the aura system are potentially empowering. Asymmetrical designs such as irregular globs are often smoky in coloration and tend to constrict the aura and suppress its energies. Many aura experts hold that these patterns can literally trap aura energies and limit positive interactions with other aura systems. When present in the aura, they usually appear in the aura's middle or lower regions where they produce a dulling effect on the surrounding energy field.

Although the origin of asymmetrical designs in the aura is unknown, many experienced aura viewers believe they are karmic in nature, particularly when their existence in the aura is long-term. Our studies found that phobias with past-life histories often appear as grayish asymmetrical designs of trapped energy in the aura. A student, whose aura signature included a grayish lump of energy, was hounded by a persistent fear of crowds which he believed to be past-life related. Through past-life regression, he discovered the source of his fear—a public execution during the French Revolution. Given insight into the past-life origin of his phobia, he assumed command of his fear and overcame it, whereupon the grayish lump and surrounding discoloration in his aura promptly vanished.

Another energy phenomenon frequently found in the aura is the so-called halo effect which, rather than a ring of energy, is actually a thin orb of intensely bright energy enveloping the aura's total external boundary. As a perimeter of intense energy, the halo's primary function is believed to be that of protection. It conserves the aura's power supply by preventing depletion from external sources which could, otherwise, drain the aura of its energy. Although the halo is valuable in sustaining the aura, it may, at the same time, limit our capacity to achieve important goals, particularly those requiring a massive expenditure of energy. Also, with the halo in place, our capacity to interact with others can become somewhat limited. Ideally, we should be able to generate the halo effect as needed, such as when the aura system is under attack, and to cancel it when its functions are no longer required. As we will discover in a later chapter, procedures have been developed to do just that.

With sufficient practice, we can each acquire skill in identifying the aura's signature characteristics, and more importantly, recognizing the empowerment relevance of each characteristic. As already emphasized, the aura's coloration and structure can provide important information of psychic significance. Among the many familiar examples are gray coloration, which often foretells adversity and disruptions in energy patterns that suggest inner turbulence. But aside from the many direct psychic indicators often appearing in the aura, the aura can provide a three-dimensional focal point that can stimulate our psychic faculties to generate relevant insight. Even among beginning viewers, clairvoyant and precognitive impressions are common during their viewings. These impressions, which can involve critical issues of life and death, often emerge as meaningful images during aura viewings.

It has been argued that the signature characteristics of the aura, including distinguishing geometric patterns, are most probably the product of the creative aura viewer. Controverting that argument is the fact that, in the experimental laboratory as well as in casual group viewing situations, highly specific aura designs, such as the pyramid and sphere, are often seen collectively and simultaneously by participating viewers. Furthermore, the designs' exact characteristics, including size, location, and coloration, are usually noted during the observations, thus suggesting something beyond chance or imagination.

Electrophotography

In addition to direct viewing strategies, various experimental procedures have been developed to study the human aura and analyze its signature characteristics. One of the most extensively researched of these procedures is electrophotography, also known as Kirlian photography and corona-discharge photography. Through this procedure, a corona-discharge is made to occur around the specimen—typically the subject's fingerpad. The specimen being photographed is placed against film, with the film situated on a dielectric positioned on a charged metal plate. The result is a photographic recording of a corona discharge or light-emitting transference of electrical charge.

In our studies, subjective inspection as well as statistical analysis of the electrophotographic recordings for hundreds of subjects revealed unique but highly stable patterns of corona-discharge activity for each individual. In a twelve-month study funded by the U. S. Army Missile Research and Development Command, the repeated fingerpad recordings for scores of experimental subjects revealed wide ranging differences among subjects but stability in pattern activity for each individual subject. Although no two recordings were ever identical, certain unique corona-discharge characteristics tended to recur at specific locations in repeated recordings for the same individual, a finding that suggests corona-discharge images could be used for identification purposes.

A later study for the Parapsychology Foundation of New York confirmed our earlier findings concerning corona-discharge pattern stability in the normal (or no-treatment) state of awareness. But when certain altered states were introduced, the study revealed significant accompanying changes in corona-discharge activity. The out-of-body state, for instance, introduced a distinct separation in the corona-discharge pattern surrounding the fingerpad, a phenomenon we called broken-corona effect, which continued for the duration of the out-of-body experience. The past-life regression state, on the other hand, produced a radiant glow in the image, a phenomenon we called past-life illumination which also continued for the duration of the altered state. These findings suggested that electrophotography could be effectively applied, not only to monitor certain altered states, but to evaluate procedures designed to induce them.

Although electrophotography is sometimes called *aura photography*, our limited studies involving only the right index fingerpad failed to validate the procedure's capacity to accurately depict the aura. Nevertheless, the corona-discharge around the right index fingerpad was found to provide, in miniature, a model which was reasonably representative of the subject's total aura. For instance, identifying characteristics such as voids and asymmetry, if found in the fingerpad recordings, were almost invariably observed elsewhere in the aura through direct viewing procedures. Figures 2 and 3 illustrate the wide range of identifying patterns noted in the electrophotographic recordings.

Our research concerning the relevance of corona-discharge photography to altered states and the human aura required highly controlled conditions in which the subject's finger orientation and the

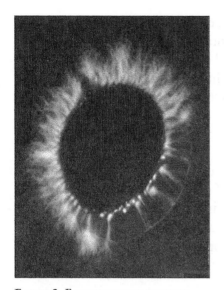

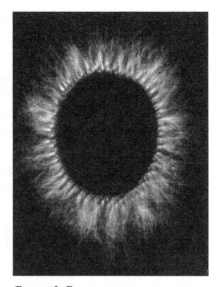

FIGURE 2. ELECTROPHOTOGRAPHIC
RECORDING, 22-YEAR-OLD MALE
COLLEGE STUDENT.
Note particularly the asymmetrical
pattern and unique arrangement of
streamers, voids, and arcs, each of
which was noted elsewhere in his
aura when it was viewed directly.

FIGURE 3. ELECTROPHOTOGRAPHIC
RECORDING, 19-YEAR-OLD FEMALE
COLLEGE STUDENT.
Note the highly symmetrical streamer
activity, a pattern which was noted
throughout her aura when it was
viewed directly.

pressure of the finger against the film were carefully controlled. The
results were repeatability and stability of the corona-discharge
images (See *Astral Projection and Psychic Empowerment* for illus-
trations of the laboratory arrangement).

In our studies, electrophotography did not provide a reliable measure of aura coloration. The color characteristics in repeated recordings for a given individual varied widely, depending on the type of
film we used.

Aura Frequency Patterns

The energy frequencies emitted by the aura provide a useful index
into the nature of the aura system. The aura frequency pattern, like
the aura itself, is developmental in nature and subject to change; nev-

ertheless it exists within an established aura structure and is thus relatively stable. Fortunately, intervention strategies that empower the aura typically generate proportional changes in aura frequencies.

Aura frequency patterns range in levels from a low of one to a high of seven, with seven representing the most refined, highly advanced frequency level. Although lower frequencies suggest a less fully developed aura system, they in no way suggest fewer growth potentials.

The distribution of aura frequency levels in the general population is similar to the distribution of many other human characteristics, with approximately two-thirds of the population showing a frequency level within an average range of three through five. Less than one percent of the general population will show an extreme frequency level of either one or seven.

The Aura Caress

Determining the aura's frequency level requires skill in first viewing the aura and practice in assessing its energy patterns. Breaks, voids, fissures, discoloration, constrictions, and asymmetry in the aura usually characterize the lower energy patterns. The effects of these and other disruptive conditions on aura frequencies can be directly assessed through a strategy known as the Aura Caress. Here is the procedure which combines visual, sensory, and subjective impressions to determine the aura's frequency level.

Step 1. Aura Viewing. View the aura and note its unique characteristics. Pay particular attention to frequency-related aspects, such as symmetry, coloration, magnitude, and brightness. Note any disruptions in the aura's patterns, including voids, fissures, discoloration, constrictions, and imbalance.

Step 2. Aura Caress. With the wrist of your subject resting lightly in the palm of your hand, sense the vibrational patterns of the aura, including intensity, harmony, and resonance. Note any interruption, sometimes called frequency static, in the flow or intensity of energy.

Step 3. Aura Scan. As your subject's wrist continues to rest in your palm, close your eyes and mentally scan your subject's aura from the head downward. Relate the scan to the subject's total aura as viewed in Step 1, noting particularly the distribution of energy patterns.

Step 4. Frequency Level. Sense again the frequency pattern being registered in your palm. Conclude the procedure by envisioning a seven-point scale with the frequency level of your subject clearly indicated.

The Aura Caress can be adapted to gauge the frequency level of oneself as well as others. Since the procedure includes several subjective elements, caress results should be considered somewhat tentative in the absence of experience or until validated by aura specialists with experience using the procedure. Only through practice can the aura's frequency characteristics be accurately determined.

Interpretation of Aura Caress results should focus on strengths and potentials rather than weaknesses and deficiencies. Typically, individuals whose aura frequency levels are low possess abundant but undeveloped potentials. Interpretation of the caress should emphasize the unlimited possibilities for continued growth, and where possible, suggest relevant empowerment strategies and growth options. In self-assessment, attention should likewise be focused on possibilities, including our capacity to use our strengths to compensate for our weaknesses.

Extra-Aura Energy Forms

Strange as it may seem to some, concentrated forms of bright energy similar to those observed in the aura are sometimes seen in settings outside the aura system. Typically appearing as glowing spheres of energy, these forms, along with apparitions as discussed in a previous chapter, are often seen as higher plane energies or else manifestations of discarnate survival, particularly when they are observed in purportedly "haunted" settings. A case in point is Brown Hall, a

Greek-Revival structure on the campus of Athens State University, Alabama (Figure 4). Over many years, an iridescent sphere of bright green energy periodically appeared at a second floor window over the building's front balcony. Though it typically appeared at night, the glow was so intense that it was occasionally visible during daylight hours.

Intrigued by the frequent reports of sightings, many of them collective in nature, a group of the students enrolled in the school's experimental parapsychology program decided to investigate the phenomenon. Equipped with various recording devices, the group assembled late in the evening at the site of the manifestation. Almost immediately, an iridescent sphere of energy appeared over a center table in the semi-darkened room. Temperature probes of the sphere revealed a Fahrenheit measurement of approximately twenty degrees greater than that of the surrounding room temperature. Unfortunately, photographic efforts to record the sphere were unsuccessful. Since the radiant green coloration of the sphere suggested healing

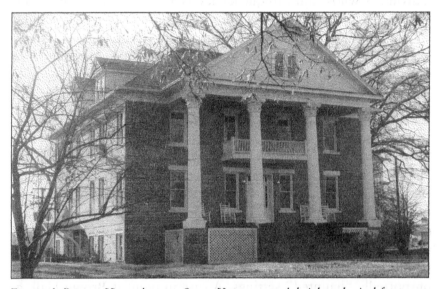

FIGURE 4. BROWN HALL, ATHENS STATE UNIVERSITY. A bright spherical form was often seen at the window over the building's front balcony *(Photo by Patricia A. Howell).*

potentials, a student with a wrist injury placed her hand in the sphere and, by her report, experienced an instant warmth throughout her body. By the end of the session, the pain and swelling in her wrist had vanished.

Following the session, the sphere became widely known for its healing qualities. Exposure to the energy form, which we called spherical therapy, proved effective in alleviating a wide range of symptoms associated with conditions such as arthritis, migraine headaches, tendinitis, and eczema, to name but a few. The sphere demonstrated unusual effectiveness in alleviating pain. A student with chronic back pain resulting from an injury experienced instant relief upon placing his hands in the sphere. Following a series of daily sessions, he fully recovered from the condition that had plagued him for several years. In another instance, a professor with a long history of inner ear problems experienced dramatic improvement upon placing his hands in the sphere. Unfortunately, the Brown Hall phenomenon with a history of over 75 years ceased when the building was recently renovated.

Energy manifestations as illustrated by the Brown Hall phenomenon have relevance to our study of the human aura in several ways. They reveal other powerful dimensions of energy and our capacity of to interact with them. They suggest a higher cosmic realm of power with purposeful energy manifestations. More importantly, they affirm the cosmic nature of our own energies.

5

Aura Empowerment Strategies

A mighty flame followeth a tiny spark.

—Dante, "Paradiso," *The Divine Comedy*
(c. 1300–21)

A S WE HAVE seen, the human aura system is more than simply an external phenomenon with features and designs holding little or no relevance to our personal empowerment. It is a fundamental force that is essential to our existence and growth. Here is a brief summary of the multiple roles of the human aura system:

- *It is a highly complex system that generates energy and sustains us mentally, physically, and spiritually.*

- *It is a sensitive yet dynamic force that encodes the totality of our individuality and connects us to the cosmic origins of our existence.*

- *It is an evolving chronicle of our past, present, and future.*

- *It is an interactive link between our innermost self and the external environment, including the aura systems of others.*

- *It is a repository of abundant resources with potential to enrich our lives.*

- *As an interactive phenomenon, it is receptive to our intervention and empowerment efforts.*

- *At any given moment, the aura is a weathervane of our personal development.*

- *The more we learn about the aura, the better we understand ourselves.*

The complex nature of the aura, rather than discouraging our study, compels us to investigate its many functions and explore its relevance to our lives. It challenges us to use our resources and technology to uncover its secrets and develop its abundant capacities.

Perhaps more than any other single human attribute, the aura reflects the true nature of our existence. As human beings, we are constantly evolving and becoming. From the psychic empowerment perspective, the skills required for viewing and interpreting the aura are critical to our growth, but they are primarily preparatory. Having acquired these basic foundation skills as presented in the preceding chapters, we are now prepared to advance to the next level of personal empowerment: deliberately interacting with the aura system, activating its capacities, and using its resources to enrich and empower our lives. Achieving these goals requires a repertoire of totally new procedures that we call aura empowerment strategies.

Aura empowerment strategies can be either general or specialized. General procedures are designed to produce an overall empowerment effect. They typically focus on the totality of our being—mentally, physically, and spiritually. Specialized procedures, on the other hand, are structured to achieve highly specific goals by focusing on a particular aura function or characteristic.

Notwithstanding their differences in design and focus, both general and specialized aura empowerment procedures have at least four common elements:

1. The application of a single empowerment procedure, whether general or specialized, tends to generate a holistic effect on the total aura system. Our studies found that even the most highly focused procedure can produce certain widespread effects, and vice versa.

2. All aura empowerment procedures are built on the human capacity for growth and change.

3. A repertoire of strategies, rather than a single procedure, is required if we are to fully maximize the aura's empowerment capacities.

4. Practice and experience are essential to the success of any empowerment strategy.

The interactive nature of the mind, body, and spirit provides the basic premise for all aura empowerment efforts. Because of its high sensitivity, the aura responds to even minute changes in the self. Deliberately inducing change, whether mental or physical, can have a profound, though often indirect, effect on the aura. For instance, procedures that relax the physical body tend to energize and expand the aura. Similarly, positive thoughts generate positive energy that can permeate the total aura system. It would follow that procedures that combine positive mental and physical elements could produce an even greater empowering effect on the human aura. The aura empowerment strategies that follow are based largely on that important concept.

The Comprehensive Intervention Procedure

The Comprehensive Intervention Procedure is a structured self-empowerment strategy that uses physical relaxation, mental imagery, and positive affirmations to infuse the aura with powerful energy. For comparison purposes, the procedure includes a "before and after" viewing of the aura. It introduces specific techniques designed to generate a fully energized mental, physical, and spiritual state that, in turn, energizes the aura. It culminates with forceful affirmations of success and well-being. The procedure can be supplemented with techniques related to specific goals, such as breaking unwanted habits, managing stress, or succeeding at an important task.

Here is the procedure, which usually requires about thirty minutes:

Step 1. Aura Preview. Find a quiet, comfortable place, and view your aura using any of the self-viewing procedures previously discussed.

Step 2. Body Scan. Settle back into a reclining or prone position, and clear your mind of all active thought. With your eyes closed, induce a deeply relaxed state by mentally scanning your physical body from the upper region down. Identify and release any accumulation of tension. Complete the body scan by taking in three deep breaths and exhaling slowly. Tell yourself after the third breath, "I am now fully relaxed."

Step 3. Energizing Imagery. Envision a powerful glow emanating from deep within yourself and slowly infusing your total body with refreshing energy. Feel the warm, invigorating energy in your central body region gently spreading in all directions, enveloping your total body in a luminous glow of energy.

Step 4. Energy Infusion. Take a few moments to allow the infusion of powerful energy to reach its peak. Focus on particular body regions, such as specific joints or small muscle groups, and notice the deep infusion of energy. Should a point of weakness or tension remain, think of it as a discoloration, then promptly replace it with the revitalizing glow of energy.

Step 5. Affirmation. As your remain relaxed and energized, affirm: *My total being—mentally, spiritually, and physically—is fully infused with powerful, positive energy. I am enveloped in the light of love, peace, and power.* Specify your goals and envision them as realities. Affirm your power to succeed.

Step 6. Aura Post-view. Conclude the procedure by again viewing your aura using the same procedure you used in Step l. Note the changes in your aura.

Comparisons of the aura before and after this procedure typically reveal a dramatic increase in both expansiveness and brightness. Although designed primarily to energize the aura, the procedure is an excellent stress management strategy. When practiced routinely, it has been highly successful in combating despondency and extinguishing many common stress-related symptoms, including fatigue, sleep disturbances, and irritability. Because it recognizes our inner capacity to take charge of the forces that influence our lives, the procedure builds self-esteem and generates powerful feelings of self-worth, both of which are critical to our personal well-being. This procedure is particularly effective in helping to achieve goals. Step 5 of the procedure is deliberately designed for that purpose. From quitting smoking to career advancement, this step sets the stage for success. When the empowerment goal, along with relevant images, are formulated, and powerful affirmations of success are factually stated, the result is a success orientation that simply cannot fail. College students have used the procedure to raise their grade-point averages, gain admission to graduate programs, and eventually get the jobs they want. In the job setting, the procedure can be used to accelerate advancement, and solve a wide range of job-related problems.

With this procedure, even distant, improbable goals become reasonable expectations. The immediate energizing effects of the procedure as reflected in the aura provide tangible confirmation of the long-range possibilities.

The Cosmic Centering Procedure

As human beings, our endless presence in the universe is not by accident, but by design. We exist within a multi-dimensional cosmic scheme which includes higher planes of energy that reach beyond the limits of time, space, and matter. But, all too often, we become disconnected from our higher self and alienated from the higher cosmic realms of power. We lose sight of the limitless potentials within ourselves and the abundant opportunities around us. Our growth gets interrupted, and eventually, we get caught in a downward spiral of hopelessness as our lives spin increasingly out of control.

Fortunately, we can re-connect to the highest sources of power—both within ourselves and beyond. The psychic empowerment concept reminds us that we can reverse the overwhelming currents that sweep us toward mediocrity and despair. We can uncover the rich resources available to us at any moment in time. We can regain the thrill of self-discovery and self-empowerment. We can experience new hope, peace, and power in our lives.

The Cosmic Centering Procedure is a self-empowerment strategy based on our capacity for oneness within ourselves and with the universe. The procedure recognizes two major sources of power: One centered in the higher part of the self and the other centered in the higher part of the cosmos. Through cosmic centering, we can become intimately connected to both. The result is an empowered state of total inner and outer attunement. The procedure holds that full empowerment is possible only when we are cosmically centered, balanced, and attuned to all the inner and outer sources of power available to us.

The procedure begins and ends with a self-viewing of the aura for comparison purposes. Approximately thirty minutes should be set aside for the procedure which is conducted in a comfortable setting free of interruptions. For this procedure, a reclining or prone position is recommended, with the legs uncrossed and hands resting comfortably to the sides.

Step 1. Aura Preview. View your aura using any of the self-viewing procedures detailed previously. Notice the specific features of your aura, including coloration, brightness, and expansiveness.

Step 2. Physical Relaxation. While resting comfortably, closed your eyes and focus only on your breathing. As you breathe deeply and rhythmically, let yourself become progressively relaxed. Take a few moments to envision a peaceful scene, such as a billowy cloud gently drifting in the breeze against a clear blue sky, and then affirm: *I am at peace with myself and the cosmos.*

Step 3. Inner Awareness. Center your full attention on the innermost part of your self. Visualize a luminous, inner core situated in your solar plexus. Think of it as an energy powerhouse radiating abundant energy that fuels your total being—mental, physical, and spiritual.

Step 4. Energy Infusion. Notice the forceful infusion of resplendent energy. Visualize your body enveloped in a radiant glow, and affirm: *I am infused with powerful, radiant energy.*

Step 5. Cosmic Imagery. Envision the distant center of the cosmos as a brilliant core of powerful energy. Think of that core as the cosmic powerhouse that fuels the universe. Focus your full attention on its limitless power.

Step 6. Cosmic Empowerment. Picture a powerful channel of bright light connecting the luminous core of your inner being to the brilliant core of the outer cosmos. As you continue to picture the gleaming shaft of pure light, let yourself become fully infused with pure cosmic energy. Affirm: *I am attuned to the cosmos and empowered with abundant cosmic energy. I am fully energized and balanced mentally, physically, and spiritually.*

Step 7. Aura Post-view. Conclude the procedure by again viewing your aura, noting particularly any changes in coloration and intensity.

In addition to its balancing and centering effects, the Cosmic Centering Procedure can be easily adapted as a strategy to unleash our creative potentials and generate totally new insight. For that application, Step 6 of the procedure is expanded to include relevant affirmations such as the following: *I am attuned to the inner and outer sources of creative power; my creative capacities are now unleashed.* Adequate time is then allowed for creative concepts, images, and ideas to emerge. Painters, sculptors, designers, architects, and writers who have experimented with this procedure attest to its effectiveness in stimulating creativity. They have discovered that just a few moments invested in this procedure can inspire creative thinking and bring forth an amazing array of creative results.

In the academic setting, the Cosmic Centering Procedure has been effective in motivating students and promoting achievement at various academic levels. Rapid progress was noted among college students participating in remedial programs when the procedure was introduced as an enrichment activity. Similar results were noted for students enrolled in advanced courses. It is conceivable that cognitive development at any academic level could be appreciably accelerated through cosmic centering techniques.

The Cosmic Centering Procedure has shown unusual promise as a psychic development strategy. Important psychic insight, particularly concerning the future, often emerges during the procedure. Because of its spontaneity in stimulating psychic awareness and accessing psychic knowledge, the procedure is often seen as the ultimate channeling phenomenon in which we experience firsthand the highest cosmic sources of insight and power.

The Aura Massage

The aura massage is an intervention procedure which involves an energy interaction between two aura systems—that of the massage specialist and subject. The procedure uses hand-massage techniques applied a few inches away from the subject's body, with palms typically turned toward the subject while carefully avoiding all physical touch. Any physical contact during the massage can interrupt the energy interaction and neutralize the empowering effects on the massage.

The aura massage is based on the concept that the aura system, while ingenuously designed and typically functional, can become impaired and inefficient. Although the aura system, like the mind and body, is endowed with a wide array of adaptive and repair mechanisms, the flow of its energy can become blocked and its empowering functions interrupted by a host of factors. Common examples are chronic stress, overwhelming adversity, unsupportive relationships, physical illness, emotional upheaval, inner conflicts, unsatisfied strivings, and a range of external influences that can be so subtle that we are unaware of their existence. Fortunately, the enfeebling consequences of these conditions on the mind, body, and spirit are usually visible in the aura, thus providing a functional context within which intervention can take place.

As an intervention procedure, the aura massage is expressly designed to empower the aura system by maximizing its functional capacities. It fortifies the aura's adaptive processes while promoting balance in the system. It can target damaged or dysfunctional regions and activate the recovery process. It can restore lost functions and revitalize the deficient aura system.

Although originally conceived as a remediation procedure, the aura massage is equally valued today for its capacity to enrich the healthy, functional aura. The massage can exercise the aura's interactive functions and introduce totally new growth options. It can gather existing aura energies and re-direct them toward designated goals. It can produce a synergistic effect by blending the energies of the mind, body, and spirit and distributing them as needed throughout the aura system.

There is mounting evidence to suggest that the aura massage can effectively promote health and fitness. As a preventive procedure, the aura massage when routinely applied is believed to build resistance to illness by fortifying the body's immune system, and there is strong evidence to suggest that it can literally accelerate the healing process. Equally as important are the palliative effects of the massage. It can enrich the lives of persons who are chronically ill or mentally distressed. As a pain management strategy, it can reduce the intensity of pain, and in some instances, extinguish pain altogether. Increasingly, enlightened health specialists in a variety of settings are using the aura massage routinely for its comforting and healing effects. The massage can target dysfunctional organs or damaged tissue and literally infuse them with bright, healthful energy. Many of the massage procedures that follow can be easily adapted to meet designated health and fitness goals.

The aura massage is more than a mechanical manipulation of another person's aura. Although the massage involves no physical touch, it can generate a powerful energy interaction between the two aura systems. While the massage specialist deliberately manages the massage within the framework of designated goals, certain spontaneous effects, including a dynamic transfer of aura energy, typically unfold. The result is a mutually empowering interchange that exercises the positive, creative capacities of both aura systems.

The essential pre-requisites for the aura massage are a receptive subject and a skilled massage specialist with a functional aura system. The massage specialist must possess an abundance of aura energy, and a genuine regard for the massage subject as a person of dignity and worth. The massage is preceded by a careful orientation in which a positive relationship with the subject is established and the goals of the massage are mutually formulated. The typical massage is accompanied by positive affirmations that maintain a productive interaction with the subject for the duration of the procedure. The massage is usually concluded with a discussion and evaluation of the massage experience.

The aura massage can be either general or specialized in nature. The general aura massage focuses on the total aura system, whereas the specialized massage focuses on a particular region of the aura or on a highly specific empowerment objective. In practice, however, the typical aura massage will include both general and specialized components. The general massage will almost always identify specific aura needs and introduce strategies to meet those needs. Similarly, the specialized aura massage will usually go beyond its specific objectives and conclude with general procedures that energize the total aura.

It is important to emphasize that nothing is more critical to the successful aura massage, whether general or specialized, than a positive interaction with the subject accompanied by relevant affirmations throughout the procedure. Suitable affirmations presented at strategic points during the massage generate powerful feelings of self-worth, and a strong, positive expectancy effect. Whether to empower the total aura or to meet highly specific aura needs, positive affirmations tend to extinguish any resistance to the massage while unleashing powerful new growth energies.

Approximately thirty minutes should be allowed for the typical massage. The physical setting should be quiet and comfortable. The massage subject can be either standing or resting comfortably in a seated or reclining position.

The General Aura Massage

The General Aura Massage is empowering in two ways: it unleashes an abundant supply of energy into the subject's total aura system, and it sets the stage for the more specialized massage strategies that are tailored to meet highly specific aura needs. Here is the eight-step procedure:

Step 1. Orientation. Although essentially preliminary in nature, this critical step determines the success or failure of the general massage. With your subject at ease in a standing, seated, or reclining position, explain the nature of the massage and its potential benefits. Involve your subject in the discussion, and candidly address any concerns or questions that may arise. Jointly formulate with your subject the goals of the massage in a permissive, non-evaluative manner.

Step 2. Self-infusement. Take a few moments to clear your mind and empower your own aura system with positive energy. Envision your aura glowing with abundant energy as you silently affirm: *My total being is infused with abundant energy. Mentally, physically, and spiritually, I am balance and attuned. I will remain fully energized throughout this exercise.*

Step 3. Subject Receptivity. Induce a receptive, relaxed state in your subject using supportive, person-centered suggestions, such as the following: *Give yourself permission to become more comfortable and relaxed. Let peace and tranquillity infuse your total being. Remind yourself that you have abundant inner potential. You are now poised for new growth and fulfillment.* Use additional positive affirmations as needed throughout the massage.

Step 4. Pre-massage Aura Viewing. View your subject's aura, noting such characteristics as coloration, magnitude, and unusual patterns. Note both deficiencies and strengths in the aura, paying particular attention to dysfunctional or weak areas. Discuss your observations with your subject in a positive, supportive manner. Additional aura viewings can be interjected as needed in the remaining steps of the procedure. Although some advanced massage specialists continuously view the aura for the duration of the massage, periodic viewing is usually sufficient to assess the effects of the massage.

Step 5. The Circular Massage. Once the initial viewing is complete, start the actual massage with gentle, circular hand motions designed to strengthen the aura and soothe areas of turbulence. Beginning at the head region, and with your palms always turned toward your subject, gently work your way downward, using slow circular motions. Avoid physical contact with your subject as your hands work together in any combination of clockwise or counter-clockwise motions.

Step 6. The Vertical Massage. Upon completion of the circular massage, use the vertical massage to evenly distribute aura energies and further soothe aura disturbances. Like the circular massage, the vertical massage begins at the head region and progresses downward. With the palms turned toward the subject, it uses slow, downward vertical strokes that end with a brisk, outward sweep of the hands. Throughout this step, attention can be focus on specific aura characteristics, including deficiencies and problem areas. Any of the more highly specialized strategies that are discussed later in this chapter can then be immediately applied, or they can be later introduced as follow-up strategies. Many massage specialists prefer postponing the specialized massage in order to gather other important information that could be useful in targeting specific needs and selecting appropriate specialized strategies.

Step 7. Post-massage Aura Viewing. With the massage now complete, again view your subject's aura. Although you probably assessed the effects of the massage on the aura as they occurred during the massage, note the overall results as seen throughout the aura system.

Step 8. Post-massage Interaction. The purpose of this final step is to review the massage experience and evaluate its results with your subject. This step usually includes a discussion of the observable changes in the subject's aura resulting from the massage. It is important to remember, however, that the best evaluation of the aura massage is the subject's self-evaluation. This step, consequently, focuses on the subject's feelings, impressions, and reactions to the experience. To complement the evaluation process, experienced massage specialists will sometimes introduce aura self-viewing strategies at this stage. The procedure is concluded with supportive comments and, whenever possible, optimistic forecasts concerning the subject's expressed goals.

It is important to keep in mind that observable characteristics in the aura are often manifestations of a deeper, internal condition. Many of the weaknesses and dysfunctions seen in the aura arise from repressed experiences that, while lost from conscious awareness, continue to function in the subconscious. Because we often have limited knowledge concerning the subject's background and history, it is important to remain psychically responsive and attuned for the duration of the massage. As our energies interact with those of the subject, essential psychic insight will often emerge. Although the aura massage does not require extensive psychical or analytical knowledge concerning the subject, we are more effective in selecting and applying the appropriate massage technique when we are aware of the aura's unseen dynamics. Knowledge of the subconscious origins of a disturbance in the aura can give rise to relevant affirmations that directly engage the subconscious. Examples of appropriate affirmations are: *As your aura becomes energized and balanced, you are also becoming energized and balanced inwardly. Even your deepest subconscious is responsive to the powerful energies of your aura.* Other positive affirmations related to more specific internal conditions can then be presented.

In many instances, aberrations or impairments in the aura are directly related to the subject's past-life experiences. The human aura is a developmental phenomenon with an extensive past-life history. Many of our conflicts and fears are known to have originated in past-life experiences that were so intense that their effects were projected into the aura and propelled into future lives. Familiar examples are the blockages and fixations in the aura that result from past-life trauma. These conditions are counteracted by insight into relevant past-life sources, and may require techniques beyond the aura massage. Past-life regression through hypnosis and the more advanced regression strategies using astral travel are particularly useful in uncovering past-life influences on the aura. (See *Astral Projection and Psychic Empowerment* for a detailed discussion of past-life regression through the out-of-body experience.)

A deeper understanding of the past-life origins of particular aura characteristics can dramatically help the general massage while suggesting specialized strategies, including affirmations that focus on not only the symptom but also the source. In instances of past-life influences, affirmations such as the following are recommended: *As your aura becomes energized, you are becoming receptive to insight from your distant past. Self-knowledge is self-power. Knowledge of your past will help you in the present to activate your inner resources and achieve your highest goals.* These somewhat general affirmations can then be supplemented with more specific affirmations related to a particular aura characteristic and its past-life source.

The Specialized Aura Massage

As noted previously, specialized massage procedures can be introduced during the general massage, or they can be implemented as an independent strategy. The focus of the specialized massage is two-fold: enriching specific aura functions, and remedying specific deficiencies or dysfunctions. Attentiveness and sensitivity throughout the massage, including intuitive awareness and psychic insight, are essential to our understanding of the subject's specialized needs, and to our success in meeting those needs.

As with other aura empowerment strategies, the specialized massage requires skill in viewing the aura, identifying particular aura needs, selecting appropriate intervention procedures, and effectively applying them. Whether to energize the "washed-out aura," repair the injured aura, induce flexibility in the rigid aura, or add color and brightness to the deficient aura, specialized procedures require precision in targeting the appropriate intervention effort. Only through practice and experience can we acquire the specialized massage skills required for effective intervention into the aura's multiple functions.

The Aura Body-Building Massage

The aura's energies can become weak and unevenly distributed, usually because of either stress or neglect of one's mental, physical, or spiritual needs. Specific areas of deficiency are usually visible either as depressions in the aura's outer edge or as "washed out" regions with weak coloration and less brightness than the surrounding areas. Like physical body-building, specialized aura body-building strategies are designed to remediate deficiencies by exercising the aura's power capacities. In aura body-building, areas of weakness are strengthened by stimulating the surrounding aura and specifically energizing the affected area.

The Aura Body-building Massage as a specialized procedure is usually implemented after the general aura massage. It begins with diagnostic viewing followed by the conventional circular hand-massage around the observed area of weakness in order to bring coloration from the surrounding area into the weak region. After a few moments of conventional circular massage, the direction of hand motion is reversed to bring brightness into the aura. The procedure then introduces the conventional vertical massage, but centering it only on the area of weakness and its immediate surroundings. The massage is concluded by briefly massaging the total aura with circular, followed by vertical, motions.

Throughout the Aura Body-building Massage, the procedure is accompanied by appropriate affirmations such as: *Your aura is becoming strong and energized. Areas of weakness in your aura are being fortified and revitalized. Bright, powerful energy is now flowing throughout your total aura system.*

In many gym settings, the Aura Body-building Massage has been effectively integrated into traditional body-building programs with amazing results. It dramatically increases motivation, self-confidence, and physical endurance. The procedure demonstrated similar effects when introduced into various sports training programs. It rapidly accelerates the development of athletic skills and improves both individual and team performance in such wide-ranging activities as wrestling, gymnastics, volleyball, golf, soccer, and archery. Male and female athletes of all ages are usually responsive to this procedure.

The Aura Repair Massage

The human aura system is vulnerable to injury, not only from the onslaught of external influences but from potentially damaging forces existing within the self. Although the aura, like the physical body, is endowed with a resilient defense system, unsuspected negative forces can target our weaknesses, launch a surprise attack against us, and penetrate our best armor.

Our strongest protection against damage to the aura is an empowered energy system with effective defenses. But even with this protection in place, damage to the aura can still occur. Among the common examples are: (a) fissures in the aura which often result from betrayal or other damaging relationships, and (b) points of darkness which suggest either vulnerability or a previous attack on the aura system from an outside source.

Fissures indicate very serious damage to the aura's essential structure. If unattended, the fissure can progressively worsen until its effects are seen throughout the aura as either enfeebling discoloration or turbulence. The location of the fissure provides an important clue to its origin. Typically, a fissure in the aura's outer region is associated with damage due to external forces, whereas, a fissure in the aura's inner region is associated with internal influences that interrupt the aura's functions.

Unlike fissures that occur typically in the aura's border regions, points of darkness can occur anywhere in the aura. When surrounded by dull discoloration, they are associated with an external attack by another energy system that has drained the aura of its energy. In a later chapter, we will further explore this phenomenon, often called psychic vampirism.

When the aura's spontaneous defense system fails, purposeful intervention becomes essential in restoring its normal function. The Aura Repair Massage is specifically designed to repair and fortify the aura, particularly when the damage involves either fissures or points of darkness. Like other specialized strategies, the Aura Repair Massage must be adapted to the individual's characteristics and needs. Although designed to repair the damaged aura, the procedure spontaneously replenishes the depleted aura's energy supply while initiating new growth and healing processes. It is important to note that serious damage to the aura will often require supplemental efforts that focus on the development of new personal empowerment skills. Here is the four-step Aura Repair Massage:

Step 1. Diagnostic Aura Viewing. Carefully view your subject's aura, noting its unique features and specific characteristics. Inspect the aura for damage by conducting a careful three-way aura scan. First, scan the aura's outer region, noting particularly any irregularity along the outside border. Then scan the aura's innermost region, paying special attention to disruptions near the physical body. Finally, scan the full aura, noting particularly any aberration in the aura's central region. Share your findings with your subject, and explore the significance of any observed damage to the aura.

Step 2. Aura Repair Plan. Formulate a repair plan with your subject based on the results of Step 1. Here is an example of an appropriate repair plan: *We will use the aura repair massage to close an opening in your aura* (specify nature of opening and location). *We will activate a repair processes that will be felt throughout your aura system and within yourself.*

Step 3. The Repair Massage. *(A) Fissures.* For damage involving fissures, gently stroke the surrounding area using circular motions to generate a build-up of positive energy around the fissure. Explain to your subject the purpose of the procedure, and affirm: *Powerful energy is now gathering around the damage in your aura.* Next, place your hands, palm sides down, to the sides of the affected area, carefully avoiding physical touch. Slowly bring your hands together, with palm facing palm, directly over the opening. Hold that position as you affirm: *Healing energies are now merging to close the opening in your aura.* Repeat this massage procedure several times. You will sense when the opening is closed. Conclude the repair massage with the affirmation: *The opening in your aura is now closed, and the healing process is now activated. Your total being is infused with powerful energy.*

(B) Points of Darkness. For points of darkness in the aura, begin the massage with conventional circular motions at the solar plexus region and then gently move the massage toward

the opening. This circular massage procedure is repeated several times to transfer energy from the solar plexus, which usually has a high concentration of energy, to the affected area. Affirm at this stage: *Powerful energy is enveloping the area of damage in your aura.* Once you sense a sufficient concentration of energy around the opening, place either hand with palm side down directly over the area of damage and gently move it toward and away from the body in gentle pumping motions, keeping the hand in the open position and avoiding any contact with the physical body. Follow the pumping motions with gentle circular motions directly over the affected area. As the circular massage continues, affirm: *Healing energy is now filling the opening in your aura. Powerful, healing energy is now unleashed throughout your total being.*

Step 4. Conclusion. Conclude the procedure with a brief, general massage of the full aura, using both circular and vertical motions along with supportive affirmations, followed by a final viewing of the aura and a brief interaction with your subject in which the empowering goals and potential benefits of the procedure are summarized.

Although the Aura Repair Massage can effectively close fissures and dark points in the aura, it is not an instant cure. Full recovery from serious damage to the aura is usually gradual, and may require other intervention procedures, particularly when the damage involves the solar plexus region of the aura. Chronic dysfunctions in that region assert a wear-and-tear effect on the total aura system. Eventually, the aura's adaptive functions become arrested and its energies severely depleted. This condition is sometimes seen in subjects who are victims of long-term, abusive relationships. Although the aura massage can offer comfort and initiate the healing process, full recovery is usually a lengthily process that requires first and foremost, a termination to the abusive relationship.

The Aura Elasticity Massage

The Aura Elasticity Massage is designed specifically to generate sufficient flexibility in the aura to close voids and restore the aura's normal energy functions. Voids are among the most common anomalies found in the human aura. They are transparent, non-functional areas that are devoid of energy. They are usually psychological in origin, but they are maintained by the aura's inflexibility and insufficient energy to bridge them. Although voids can exist anywhere in the aura, they seem to occur with greater frequency in the upper regions. When a void is present, the full aura is often constricted due to the inelasticity that maintains the void. They are often found in the auras of persons who experience difficult interpersonal relationships, feelings of emptiness or alienation, and lack of meaning in their lives.

In addition to closing voids and restoring normal functions, the Aura Elasticity Massage is structured to replenish the total aura with an abundant supply of new energy and build the subject's awareness of dormant inner resources. Here is the procedure:

Step 1. Aura Viewing. View your subject's aura, and upon discovering a void, note specifically its location and size. Share your aura observations with your subject. Describe the void, including its shape, size, and location. Help your subject to visualize the void exactly as it appears in the aura. Non-judgmentally explore with your subject the relevance of the void.

Step 2. Goal Formulation and Orientation. With the active participation of your subject, formulate the massage goals. State them as specific, positive outcomes. Examples of appropriate goals are: *We will use the massage to generate sufficient energy and flexibility in your aura to close any existing void. Once the void is closed, you will discover new sources of power in your life. You will find new ways of enriching and empowering your life.* Orient your subject concerning the elasticity massage and its effect on voids in the aura. The effectiveness of the massage in closing voids depends to a great extent your subject's ability to visualize the void as it diminishes in size and finally vanishes.

Step 3. Spherical Massage. Begin the massage by cupping your hands, one to each side of the void, and visualizing a sphere of radiant energy between your palms fully enveloping the void and its immediate surroundings. Slowly massage the envisioned sphere, using gentle, flowing hand motions. As you bring your hands closer and closer together over the void, sense the void progressively shrinking until it finally disappears altogether. With your palms interfaced and resting at the location of the former void, affirm: *The void in your aura is now replaced with bright, vibrant energy.*

Step 3. Circular Massage. Using conventional circular motions, massage the former void region as you affirm: *With your aura now energized, you are discovering a new wealth of inner potential.* Gradually expand the circular massage to take in larger regions of the aura as your affirm: *Your aura is now empowered and fully functional. You are surrounded by unlimited opportunities for enrichment and success.* Formulate other empowering affirmations that address the specific growth needs of your subject.

Step 4. Conclusion. Again view your subject's full aura, noting particularly the balanced energy and concentrated brightness replacing the former void. End the procedure by sharing these final observations with your subject.

The Aura Color Massage

Color is one of the aura's most important components. Here is a brief summary of the role of color in the human aura:

1. Color, like other aura signature features, exists within a relatively stable aura structure.

2. Although coloration patterns vary widely, the aura is typically characterized by a dominant color along with lesser colors arranged in a variety of designs.

3. The rainbow aura consists of layers of color that can either encompass the full body or appear as a localized phenomenon, usually around the head and shoulders.

4. The relatively rare single color aura is characterized by wide variation in color intensity, with a fading of color normally noted in the outer regions of the aura.

5. The aura can accommodate transient colors which temporarily engage either the full aura or isolated regions. This phenomenon can have important mental, physical, and spiritual significance.

6. Areas of dull discoloration are usually seen as enfeebling in that they tend to impair the aura system's functional capacities, particularly in generating energy.

7. The brightness of a particular color in the aura offers an index to its empowerment functions, with the brighter the color, the more empowering its capacity.

8. Although areas of white, black, and no coloration can appear in the aura, the human aura is never totally white, black, or without color.

9. A relationship between aura coloration and other personal characteristics, including mental, physical, and spiritual, has been established. Here are a few of the colors commonly found in the human aura and some of the personal traits often associated with them:

> Blue: *Tranquillity, balance, flexibility, optimism, and when a deep hue, mental alertness and emotional control.*
>
> Yellow: *Intelligence, sociability, and dependability.*
>
> Green: *Healing and self-actualization.*
>
> Pink: *Youth, rejuvenation, sensitivity, idealism, and talent.*
>
> Brown: *Practicality, stability, outdoor interests, and independence.*
>
> Purple: *Philosophical and abstract interest.*
>
> Orange: *Extroversion and competitiveness.*
>
> Gray: *Adversity or impending misfortune.*

The Aura Color Massage has two major functions. The first, called color enrichment, enriches aura coloration by increasing the richness to existing colors. The second, called color addition, introduces totally new colors into the aura, as either a localized mass or a layer fully enveloping the aura. Both functions are based on the concept that each color in the aura represents a differential energy with unique empowerment potential. Both functions recognize the aura's capacity to generate an energy product and transfer it to another aura system in a color form. Positive affirmations along with explanations of the specific massage techniques and their purposes are interspersed throughout the procedure.

In the Aura Color Massage, color enrichment accentuates the positive traits associated with a certain color already present in the aura. The procedure selects a particular trait from those associated with a given color, and then uses appropriate strategies to introduce a bright, rich concentration of the desired color with its accompanying trait into the aura system. For instance, increasing the richness of pink in the aura can generate youthful energy, strengthen a specific talent, or exercise the subject's capacity for sensitivity, depending on the characteristic selected for emphasis. Enriching the aura with yellow, on the other hand, can increase intelligence, sociability, or dependability, again depending on the characteristic selected for emphasis. Our laboratory studies found that increasing the richness of yellow in the aura appreciably raised the IQ as measured by pre- and post-tests of intelligence, but only when the designated empowerment goal was to strengthen intellectual functions. Of particular interest were massive gains in verbal skills, which are associated not only with intelligence but also with sociability, another characteristic related, as already noted, to the color yellow.

Color addition is considered a more radical intervention procedure than color enrichment because it literally changes the aura's color composition by adding a completely new color, either as a localized region or a new layer enveloping the full aura. Although there is some evidence to suggest that each human aura may include to some extent all conceivable colors and their representative energies, the visible aura often appears entirely deficient of certain colors. The color addition technique holds that the introduction of a totally new color energy into the aura system could introduce any of the personal characteristics associated with that color. The color addition strategy is similar to color enrichment in that it first determines the desired additive from among the traits associated with different colors and then tailors the procedure to fit that additive. For instance, if the desired additive is practicality, the color brown, which is associated with that trait, would be selected for addition to the aura. On the other hand, if the desired additive is healing, bright green energy would be selected for addition, typically near the dysfunctional area. The procedure would then be specifically structured to introduce both the desired color and its related value. Although other characteristics associated with a particular color can accompany both the enrichment and additive process, the specified trait will assume dominance due primarily to the selective use of appropriate images and affirmations. It should be noted that, in most instances, the added color eventually fades from the aura, but the empowerment benefits associated with it tend to remain intact.

Here is the Aura Color Massage, including procedures for both color enrichment and color addition:

Step 1. Aura Viewing. View your subject's aura, paying particular attention to features such as deficiencies, discoloration, and other limitations that suggest a need for color enrichment or addition.

Step 2. Goal Formulation. Formulate specific massage goals, with your subject actively participating in the process. Examples include enriching an existing color to increase a particular characteristic associated with that color, or adding a new color to the aura in order to initiate a totally new function.

Step 3. Power Spin. While standing to the side of your subject who preferably is also standing, begin the color massage by generating a power spin of energy at the body's central trunk region. Use circular movements only, with one hand at the front and one hand at the back of your subject. Gradually expand the movements until they encompass the full central region of the aura. For the reclining subject, massage only the front trunk region using circular movements.

Step 4. Energy Concentration. Upon completing the power spin, rub your palms together to generate a concentration of energy between them. Whether to enrich an existing color or to add a new color to the aura, envision the desired color as bright energy builds between your hands. Separate your palms and, with the hands cupped, bring them together and apart several times to create a sphere of energy between your palms. Continue the rhythmic, to-and-fro hand movements until the sphere of concentrated energy is fully formed. At this point in the procedure, the sphere of radiant color will usually become visible between the cupped hands. Place your cupped hands holding the sphere of energy in the area of the aura to be energized.

Step 5. Color Intervention. This step introduces three intervention options: color enrichment, color addition, and color layer addition. Positive affirmations, along with appropriate explanations, are critical to each of these options.

(A) Color Enrichment. To enrich an existing color in the aura, place your cupped hands holding the sphere of energy in the area of the aura to be enriched. Release the sphere into the subject's aura by turning your palms toward your subject. Once the bright sphere is positioned, gently massage the color region with circular hand motions that concentrate first on the sphere and then slowly expand to encompass larger regions of the aura.

(B) Color Addition. To introduce a totally new color into a localized region of the aura, place the energy sphere in the center of the selected area to be energized and gently massage it into the aura using circular hand motions. For this application, the massage remains localized.

(C) Color Layer Addition. To introduce a new layer of color into the full aura, place the sphere of color in the solar plexus region of the aura and disperse the new energy by massaging the aura with gentle, circular hand motions, beginning at the solar plexus region and gradually expanding the massage to encompass the full aura. Introducing a new layer of color is an excellent procedure for protecting the aura from attack or invasion by negative forces. The recommended colors for that purpose are a bright blue for mental

protection, bright green for physical protection, and bright purple for spiritual protection.

Step 6. General Massage. Conclude the procedure with a general massage, including a combination of circular and vertical movements over the total aura system.

The empowerment implications of color enrichment and addition to the human aura are indeed profound. In a range of settings—educational, rehabilitation, correctional, medical, and psychotherapeutic—the Aura Color Massage has almost unlimited possibilities as an empowerment strategy in bringing forth positive change. It stimulates the aura's existing capacities and in some instances, introducing totally new growth resources or clusters of new power in the form of color energy. As already noted, we can literally increase intelligence by introducing yellow, slow aging by introducing pink, and accelerate healing by introducing green. Our studies found that introducing bright blue into the aura literally altered brain-wave patterns and produced the alpha state, which is associated with tranquillity and inner peace. It would seem plausible that there exists an aura color or color combination appropriate to every human striving.

As a point of caution, the aura massage must never attempt to add gray or dull discoloration to the aura. Any deliberate effort to transfer disempowering coloration or any other negative influence to another aura system is always self-damaging.

The Pain Management Aura Massage

From the psychic empowerment perspective, the goal of pain management is: (1) to reduce or eliminate pain and, (2) replace pain with healing energy. Although the pharmaceutical approach remains the conventional pain management strategy, it is not always effective. Numerous innovative approaches based on the mind/body connection have emerged, among them self-hypnosis, biofeedback, meditation, and relaxation. These procedures, which should be considered essentially supplemental to conventional approaches, recognize the power of the mind to influence biological processes, including those related to pain.

The Pain Management Aura Massage differs from other pain management procedures. It focuses on the aura as an interactive energy system with the specialized capacity to reduce or eliminate pain while attending to the underlying psychological and biological factors associated with the pain. It introduces a Pain Intensity Scale and engages the active participation of the subject in altering the level of pain. The procedure is designed for use with appropriate medical guidance. Here is the procedure:

Step 1. Pre-assessment and Goal Statement. First, review the history of your subject's pain. Determine, as far as possible, the pain's origins and dynamics. With your subject, explore the specific location and characteristics of the pain, such as dull, sharp, radiating, throbbing, burning, and so-forth. Assist your subject in rating the severity of the pain on a ten-point Pain Intensity Scale, with a rating of one indicating no pain and a rating of ten indicating severe pain (Figure 5). With the active participation of your subject, formulate the pain management objectives, which can range from total elimination of pain to reducing the pain's intensity to a more moderate level on the Pain Intensity Scale. Instruct your subject to place a second mark on the scale as the pain management goal. Orient your subject concerning pain as a physical sensation rather than a personal trait to be owned and rewarded. Refer to pain as the pain or the discomfort rather than your pain or your discomfort. Likewise, encourage your subject to refer to pain objectively, since subjective

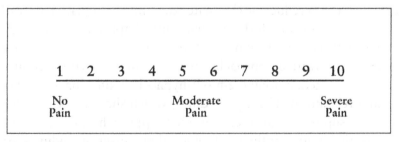

FIGURE 5. PAIN INTENSITY SCALE.
For rating the severity of pain on a scale of one-to-ten.

references such as my pain or my discomfort can promote personal ownership of pain and possible reluctance to alleviate or extinguish it.

Step 2. Aura Massage. Massage the subject's full aura from the head downward, using gentle, circular hand motions designed to evenly distribute the aura's energies and minimize turbulence which is often produced by physical pain. Accompany the massage with positive affirmations, such as: *You are becoming balanced and attuned mentally, physically, and spiritually,* then resume the circular massage but limiting it to the area of pain. As the massage continues, instruct your subject to envision the Pain Intensity Scale, with the pain level slowly falling until it reaches the desired level. Allow plenty of time for the pain intensity to subside and decline to the desired level. Once the desired level is reached, rub your palms together as you envision a concentration of luminous green energy forming in your hands. Then, hold your palms for a few moments over the affected body area as you mentally release the bright concentration to infuse your subject with comforting, healing energy.

Step 3. Supportive Affirmations. End the procedure with supportive affirmations such as the following: *You are now fully infused with powerful, comforting energy. Your inner healing resources are now unleashed to permeate your total being. You can banish any future threat of pain by envisioning yourself enveloped in radiant energy.*

This procedure can be easily revised and applied as a self administered procedure for managing pain. When adapted for self use, the full aura massage is replaced by a regional massage around the pain area. The regional massage is then gradually constricted until it is centered on the area of pain.

The Luminous Massage

The Luminous Massage is designed to infuse the total aura system with brightness and abundant energy. This is the ultimate aura massage. It is potentially empowering to the subject and massage specialist alike. In illuminating the aura, the procedure makes no attempt at aura cleansing, a misnomer since the aura never becomes unclean; more accurately, it becomes dysfunctional and inefficient. The dull, dingy, or discolored aura is not "dirty," but instead, deficient in brightness or diluted in energy.

Unlike the Color Massage, the Luminous Massage does not intervene into the aura's coloration. It is not designed to enrich existing colors or add new ones. It does not attempt to redistribute aura energy or to directly repair the damaged aura system. Its primary goal is to engage the subject in an empowerment interaction that culminates in a full infusion of luminous cosmic energy.

The Luminous Massage is somewhat mystical in nature since the massage specialist functions as an energy medium through which pure cosmic energy is channeled to the subject. In this procedure, the energies of the massage specialist are blended with the higher energies of the cosmos to generate a spherical energy form that is then transferred to the subject's aura as bright light. The subject's total aura, including voids and areas of dinginess and discoloration, is fully infused with radiant new energy. The first three steps of the procedure prepare the massage specialist for Step 4 and the literal transfer of cosmic energy to the subject. Here is the procedure:

Step 1. Inner Attunement. With your subject seated comfortably, prepare for the massage by clearing your mind of all active thought. Empty your mind of all problems, cares, and tension. Close your eyes and envision the center of your being radiating powerful energy in the form of white light in all directions, infusing and revitalizing your total energy system. Sense the vibrant energy permeating your physical body. Absorb tranquillity into every fiber of your being. Silently affirm: *My mind, body, and spirit are fully infused with the light of love, peace, and power.*

Step 2. Cosmic Attunement. As your eyes remain closed, envision the distant center of the cosmos radiating pure, white light. Turn your palms upward as you visualize radiant cosmic energy streaming into your hands and melding with your own aura system to form a powerful union of energy in its purest form. Sense the infusion of pure cosmic energy, first in your hands and then throughout your total being. Silently affirm: *Mentally, physically, and spiritually, I am infused with pure cosmic energy.*

Step 3. Energy Condensation. Cup your palms and turn them so that they face each other. Visualize a sphere of white light taking shape between your cupped hands. Gently massage the sphere until you sense its warmth and vitality. Continue to massage the developing sphere of energy as its intensity builds. You can sense the concentration of energy as it forms in your hands. The concentration of energy can be seen as a white glow when your hands are held at arm's length and attention is focused at the center-point between your cupped hands. We call this phenomenon the materialization of light.

Step 4. Energy Transfer. With the white glow of energy suspended between your hands, place your cupped hands a few inches over the head of your subject, and release the sphere by slowly separating your hands. Beginning with the glowing sphere now suspended over your subject's head, gently massage the aura with downward strokes to distribute the concentration of energy throughout the aura. Allow plenty of time for the aura to fully absorb the sphere of energy.

Step 5. Affirmation. Conclude the energy infusion process by affirming: *Your total being is now totally infused with pure radiant energy. You are enveloped in the light of love, peace, and power. Mentally, physically, and spiritually, you are attuned and energized.*

The Luminous Massage is an advanced massage procedure. Its use is recommended only after practice using other aura massage techniques. With repeated practice of this procedure, many massage experts develop skill in generating a concentrated sphere of bright luminous energy that is clearly visible to the subject as well as others who may be witnessing the massage. Even during energy transfer in

Step 4, the glowing sphere is usually visible as it remains briefly suspended over the subject's head before being gently assimilated into the full aura. Following the massage, the aura typically expands as it assumes a sparkling new brilliance, effects that are quite long-lasting. Some massage subjects describe the Luminous Massage as a peak experience that is permanently integrated into their total self.

Like the Pain Management Aura Massage, the Luminous Massage can be self-administered with only minor modifications.

The Aura Self-Massage

Positive interactions within the self, as with others, can be enlightening, energizing, and empowering. The concept of self-empowerment is based on that simple premise. We can deliberately generate positive thought messages that build self-confidence and feelings of self-worth. We can create positive mental images that empower us to achieve our personal and career goals. We can engage a powerful mind/body interaction that promotes better health and fitness. Through the aura self-massage, we can interact with our personal aura system and activate its highest empowerment capacities.

Rather than a single intervention procedure, the aura self-massage is a constellation of numerous strategies with objectives that vary from strategy to strategy. Unlike other massage procedures, the self-massage will occasionally involve physical touch but only where indicated.

The X Self-Massage

The X Self-massage is a self-energizing procedure designed to stimulate the aura system and distribute its energies more evenly. The result is an enriched and more expansive aura with many positive spin-off effects. For this procedure, a comfortable reclining or supine position is recommended.

Step 1. The X Position. Begin the X Self-massage by closing your eyes (keeping them closed for the duration of the procedure) and crossing your arms to form an X across your chest. With your arms crossed and resting against your chest, place your hands on your shoulders as you breathe slowly, deeply, and regularly. Take a few moments to relax as you clear your mind of active thought.

Step 2. Aura Imagery. While maintaining the X position, envision your full aura, noting its colors, patterns, and unique features. Give particular attention to the aura surrounding your upper body.

Step 3. Two-stage Massage. *Stage I.* As your arms remain crossed, lift your hands and arms a few inches from your body, then gently stroke the aura around your chest and shoulders, using slow circular hand motions. Envision the aura around your hands and arms interacting with the aura around your chest and shoulders. Sense the energizing effects of the massage deep within your body.

Stage II. Uncross your arms and place your hands to the sides of your head, and with your palms turned toward your temples, use circular motions to gently massage the aura, being careful to avoid all physical touch. Extend the circular hand massage by moving slowly downward to include the shoulders, chest, abdomen, and hips. Further extend the massage by using brisk, vertical motions that sweep energies from your trunk region downward. Reverse the downward direction of the massage, slowing massaging upward with circular strokes, and finally culminating at the head region.

Step 4. Self-empowerment Affirmations. Return your arms to the original crossed position and, with your hands resting on your shoulders, affirm: *I am enveloped in positive, powerful energy. I am at my peak mentally, physically, and spiritually. I am empowered to achieve my highest goals.*

The X Self-massage is a multi-purpose procedure. Students who regularly practice it report a dramatic improvement in their academic performance. When practiced immediately prior to a course evaluation, the procedure tends to stimulate clear thinking and better memory of course materials. Other benefits reported include greater self-confidence and strong feelings of security and personal worth.

In the clinical setting, the procedure has been highly effective in reducing stress and improving coping skills. It has shown particular promise as an intervention strategy when incorporated into alcohol and drug treatment programs.

When practiced regularly, it tends to build self-esteem, motivation, and a strong success orientation. The X Self-massage is also valued as a psychic protection procedure. It builds a powerful aura system that resists the intrusion of negative influences, including those involving unexpected altercations, pressures, or threats to the self. Following practice of this procedure, many subjects find that simply crossing the arms to form an X across the chest is sufficient to instantly energize the aura and protect it against any onslaught of negative forces.

The Self-Rejuvenating Massage

Although rejuvenation is an indirect spin-off of many aura massage strategies, maximizing the aura's rejuvenating capacities requires specialized procedures that focus directly on the aging process. The Self-rejuvenating Massage is specifically designed to either slow or reverse aging by activating the aura's rejuvenating energies and channeling them to designated targets.

The Self-rejuvenating Massage is based on the premise that aging is a multi-faceted, interactive phenomenon with many determinants and influencing factors. It holds that physical, psychological, and even spiritual elements converge to affect aging. By directly intervening into any one of these influences, we can alter the interaction and re-direct the aging process.

Although aging is a characteristically autonomous process, negative influences can accelerate it. Common examples are excessive stress, feelings of helplessness, smoldering hostility, unresolved conflict, and low self-esteem, all of which tend to deplete our adjustment resources, lower our resistance to disease, enfeeble our biological systems, and indirectly accelerate aging. On the other hand, a positive mental state, a healthy self-concept, a sense of humor, and an optimistic outlook are always empowering, rejuvenating, and health-enhancing.

The Self-rejuvenating Massage introduces techniques that revitalize the aura system as well as the underlying biological and psychological factors related to aging. The procedure recognizes the rejuvenating power of constructive imagery and positive affirmations. It introduces unique massage movements designed to "lift" the aura and initiate an upward flow of energy. Here is the procedure, which is usually conducted in the seated or reclining position, with your eyes closed.

Step 1. Relaxation. Slow your breathing and envision a vapor gently rising around you to envelop your total body. As the vapor slowly rises, let your body become increasingly relaxed. Affirm to yourself that the vapor signifies a higher cosmic energy force that empowers your physical body and aura system. Once your body is fully enveloped, allow the vapor to become transformed into a iridescent glow. Slowly breathe in the glow as your affirm: *I am absorbing peace and serenity throughout my total being.*

Step 2. Rejuvenation Regression. Mentally travel back in time, and envision yourself at your youthful prime, perhaps standing before a full-length mirror, disrobed and glowing with the energies of youth. Note especially the radiant glow around your body and the youthful gleam in your eyes as you affirm, *This is the true me.* Focus your attention on your solar plexus region as the rejuvenating center of your aura system. Breathe in the glow of youth surrounding your body, absorbing rejuvenating energy deeply within yourself. Affirm: *My total being is fully infused with rejuvenating energy.* Sense the energies of youth flowing throughout your body.

Step 3. Two-stage Rejuvenating Massage. *Stage I.* Massage the aura emanating from your central body region with slow, upward hand strokes that end with a gentle outward sweep. Focus first on the lower area and work your way upward using only vertical strokes and outward sweeps, while always avoiding physical contact. Envision the energies related to aging as discolorations that are being swept away from your aura system. Upon reaching the head region, continue the upward vertical movements, but let them end with gentle backward strokes to the sides of your head. Conclude this stage of the massage with the upward facial sweep, a procedure that gently strokes the aura emanating from the face, using upward hand movements that end with a backward sweep over the head while envisioning a radiant glow of rejuvenating energy around your body.

Stage II. Rub your hands gently together as you visualize rejuvenating energy in the form of bright pink light being concentrated in your palms. Again massage your aura using the procedure as detailed in Stage I, beginning at your central body region and culminating with the face massage. Envision your aura as it takes on the pink glow of youth. As you stroke the aura around your face, notice the tingling, rejuvenating sensations. Allow the muscles in your face to respond to the upward strokes by soaking in rejuvenating energy.

Step 4. Concluding Affirmations and Post-massage Cue. The goal of this step is two-fold: first, to fortify the immediate results of the massage, and second, to establish the upward facial sweep as a post-massage cue for use on command to instantly activate rejuvenation. To achieve this goal, envision your body again enveloped in radiant energy as you affirm: *My total being is revitalized and infused with rejuvenation. I will, on command, instantly activate rejuvenation by upwardly stroking the energies emanating from my face as I envision the radiant glow surrounding my body.*

The upward facial sweep as a rejuvenation cue can be used almost anywhere and as often as needed. Frequent use of this rejuvenating gesture can generate a visible glow around the face while reducing or preventing the signs of aging, including neck and facial wrinkles. Although the Self-rejuvenating Massage is a cutting-edge empowerment strategy, the upward facial sweep as an age-defying gesture is not new. At age 97, a former teacher known for her quick wit and incredibly youthful appearance reports regular use of the upward facial sweep (although she does not label it as such). While attributing her youthful appearance to the upward facial sweep, she believes her long life is due in part to the energizing influence of an emerald ring, a treasured heirloom which she wears daily. Together, the upward facial sweep, the emerald, and perhaps even more important, her remarkable sense of humor seem to empower her with the essential resources for rejuvenation and longevity. In a later chapter, we will discuss the effects of the emerald and other gems on the human aura system.

The Aura Self-Healing Massage

The physical body is a wondrously complex structure with many organs, functions, and systems, all incredibly designed to work together in perfect harmony. It can be compared to an amazing computer system that can accommodate continuous input and efficiently integrate it into a flexible, adaptive system. But like the most sophisticated computer system, the physical body is subject to power failure, overload, and glitches in its components and operations. It can be invaded by agents that contaminate the system and disrupt its functions. It may require downloading, jump-starting, or reprogramming. In severe instances, the physical body, like the computer, may literally shut down.

The Aura Self-healing Massage is designed to introduce new healing energies into the physical body, and wherever needed, to restore normal functions to specific organs and systems. It focuses on the mind, body, and spirit interaction, while emphasizing the responsiveness of each interactive component to the others. By deliberately introducing positive energy into the interaction, the procedure enriches the total system. More specifically, it transmits positive healing energy to weakened elements and operations. It empowers the total aura system with energy in its purest, brightest form. The Aura Self-healing Massage recognizes the healing power within ourselves as well as our capacity to access and interact with higher sources of healing, including spiritual dimensions and their ministering entities.

(See *Psychic Empowerment for Health & Fitness* for a further discussion of higher sources of healing energy.) The procedure requires approximately thirty minutes in a quiet, comfortable setting free of distractions.

Step 1. Physical Relaxation. Assume a comfortable seated or reclining position, and take a few deep breaths, exhaling slowly. Mentally scan your body from the head downward, pausing at points of tension as you relax every fiber, joint, and tendon. Envision relaxation as soft light accompanying the scan, slowly illuminating your entire body. Let relaxation soak into the body's innermost regions to permeate every organ and system.

Step 2. Inner Energy Infusion. With your physical body now fully relaxed, envision the bright inner core of your aura system in your solar plexus region. Sense the pulsating energy emanating from that luminous core and spreading in all directions throughout your body. Take a few moments to allow the energy infusion to reach its peak.

Step 3. Solar Plexus Aura Massage. Massage the aura in your solar plexus region with gentle circular hand motions, alternating your hands as you envision healing energy spreading outward in all directions. Follow the circular massage with vertical motions using both hands to spread the healing energy evenly into your upper and lower body. Conclude the aura massage with wide, circular motions as you envision each organ and system of your body becoming infused with bright shining energy. Envision your circulatory system aglow with healing energy, dispersing it into every fiber of your body. Allow the infusion process to reach its highest point, and then affirm: *The healing power within myself is now unleashed, permeating my total body with healing energy.*

Step 4. Cosmic Energy Infusion. Picture the center of the cosmos as a brilliant sphere of pure radiant energy. Visualize the powerful cosmic core radiating immeasurable power that sustains the universe. Think of your hands as your body's antennae with power to receive healing energy from the center of the cosmos.

Lift your hands, and with your palms turned upward, visualize streams of bright energy from the cosmic core entering your palms and uniting with the core of your own energy system, infusing and energizing it with unlimited power. Focus your attention on the inner gathering of healing energy. Allow a few moments for the cosmic infusion process to reach its peak.

Step 5. Cosmic Aura Massage. As you visualize the powerful union of energy at the core of your aura system, spread cosmic healing energy throughout your body by repeating the solar plexus aura massage described in Step 3 above, beginning with circular motions, followed by vertical motions, and ending with additional circular motions. Visualize bright cosmic energy being distributed throughout your body. Sense the vibrant renewal process in your body.

Step 6. Focused Massage. To center healing energy on any designated body regions, organ, or systems, focus the aura massage on that area using slow circular motions. Envision the target during the focused massage as it becomes infused with luminous healing energy.

Step 7. Concluding Affirmations. Conclude the procedure with relevant affirmations such as: *I am attuned mentally, physically, and spiritually to the highest sources of power. My total being is filled and overflowing with power. Physically, I am energized with health and vitality. Mentally, I am at peace. Spiritually, I am empowered by a new awareness of the supreme power within myself. I am at the pinnacle of oneness with the cosmic origin of my existence.*

Many subjects who practice this procedure experience profound spiritual enlightenment or an exciting new awareness of higher dimensions of power. In Step 4 of the procedure, spontaneous interactions with ministering angels and spirit guides often accompany the merging of cosmic energy with the aura's inner core. By simply extending Step 4, we can deliberately access higher spiritual dimensions and engage deeply meaningful interactions with these guides.

6

Hypnosis and the Human Aura

If I were to begin life again, I should want it as it was. I would only open my eyes a little more.

—Jules Renard, Journal
(March, 1906)

HYPNOSIS AS APPLIED to personal empowerment is based on a two-fold premise: first, within each of us is a vast region of fathomless growth potential, and second, through appropriate strategies, we can activate those potentials to empower and enrich our lives. From the psychic empowerment perspective, we are the totality of all that we have experienced. But much of our past lies beyond the reach of the conscious mind in that rich, uncharted region called the subconscious. Existing there, along with enormous but often dormant growth resources, are all past experiences not presently available to conscious awareness. The subconscious, by its existence alone, challenges us to probe its innermost regions and uncover its hidden wealth of knowledge and growth potential.

Hypnosis is one of the most effective empowerment tools known for accessing the subconscious and uncovering new growth possibilities. It can activate dormant potential, unblock hidden growth channels, and unleash tremendous new power in our lives. As a result, goals otherwise unattainable can become reasonable possibilities.

Hypnosis can be defined simply as a trance state in which our receptivity to suggestion is heightened. The depth of the trance can range from a mild state of increased receptivity to a profound, somnambulist-like state of altered consciousness. The light-to-moderate trance is usually sufficient for most self-empowerment purposes, including highly specific goals such as managing weight, quitting smoking, reducing stress, increasing creativity, improving memory, and accelerating the rate of learning, to list but a few. A more profound trance state is usually required for applications such as past-life regression and the recovery of painful memories buried deeply in the subconscious. Post-hypnotic suggestions can be effective at any trance depth.

There is some evidence to suggest that hypnosis can literally create certain highly complex, full-blown skills, such as the immediate command of a new language, or instant awareness of new knowledge. Because this remarkable phenomenon, which is sometimes called hypno-production, is occasionally observed during hypnotic past-life regression, it is often attributed to the awakening of dormant skills or past-life memories recorded in the subconscious.

Hypnosis can be used to uncover our psychic abilities and stimulate our psychic development. Many of our psychic potentials seem to exist in the subconscious. Because they are out of the reach of the conscious mind, they tend to surface only sporadically through subtle channels such as dreams, déjà vu, or intuitive impressions. During hypnosis, psychic manifestations often emerge spontaneously in direct, undisguised form. Among the common examples are precognition, telepathy, clairvoyance, out-of-body experiences, and past-life regression. Numerous hypnotic procedures have been formulated to exercise our psychic capacities and activate specific psychic functions. (See *Psychic Empowerment: A 7-Day Plan for Self-Development* for a detailed discussion of hypnosis as a psychic development strategy.)

In using hypnosis as a personal empowerment tool, self-hypnosis is the preferred strategy. In reality, all hypnosis is self-hypnosis since in the absence of a receptive subject, the trance state will not occur. Self-hypnosis differs from hypnosis only in that the trance state is self-induced and self-directed. Once mastered, the techniques of self-hypnosis can be used to achieve the same goals as hypnosis, and in most instances, with even greater effectiveness.

Self-hypnosis is important to our study of the human aura for several reasons. By tapping into our subconscious, self-hypnosis offers a totally new channel for viewing and interacting with the aura. It can activate those psychic faculties, including clairvoyance and psychokinesis (PK), which are especially relevant to our self-intervention efforts. It can bring forth resources submerged in the subconscious and apply them to energize the aura and empower our lives. Many subjects report seeing their full aura for the first time during the self-induced trance state. Although awareness of the aura during hypnosis is often spontaneous, it can be voluntarily produced through certain specialized trance procedures, which we will later discuss.

Self-hypnosis, of course, is only one of several techniques that enable us to see and interact with our own aura. A major advantage of self-hypnosis lies in its capacity to reveal the full aura while permitting direct intervention into its various functions. Self-viewing techniques often reveal only a partial picture of the aura, and thus provide only limited opportunities for self-intervention. A comprehensive view of the aura permits self-intervention that focuses on such singular needs as voids, fissures, and discoloration that can occur anywhere in the aura.

Once the full aura is visible through self-hypnosis, we can deliberately intervene to influence particular functions, even as we remain in the trance state. While the trance state alone is potentially rewarding, it is valued primarily as a means to an end. Through self-hypnosis, we can energize the aura, introduce changes in coloration, make adjustments in energy patterns, correct dysfunctional areas, and promote balance among functions. Of equal or even greater importance, we can use post-hypnotic suggestions to boost our aura perception, interpretation, and intervention skills.

It is important to note that the trance induction process is often accompanied by visible changes in the aura. Our studies found that the effects of the ensuing trance on the aura depend largely on the induction procedure used. The conventionally authoritative, restrictive, and demanding induction approach used by some professional hypnotists tends to constrict the subject's aura and diminish its brilliance, conditions that tend to linger for the trance's duration. These reactions are probably due to our natural tendency to resist negative influences, including the demands imposed by a dominating hypnotist. Perhaps as expected, the more permissive trance induction approaches using positive techniques, such as peaceful imagery and physical relaxation, tend to expand and illuminate the aura. Once the trance state is achieved through positive induction procedures, the aura typically resumes its normal prehypnotic state.

Whether to simply view our own aura or to intervene into its functions, a positive self-induction strategy designed to generate a light-to-moderate trance state is recommended. In some instances, a deep trance state can actually interfere in our ability to see and work with the aura. Among the numerous self-induction procedures now available, the most efficient for aura self-viewing and intervention are the Finger-spread and Peripheral Glow Methods. Both methods use permissive techniques that recognize the mind, body, and spirit interaction, as well as our capacity to deliberately influence the interaction. When properly applied, both methods are equally effective for viewing the aura and introducing moderate changes, such as enriching the aura's color and brightness. For serious intervention efforts involving radical manipulation of the aura, such as correcting fissures or filling voids, the Finger-Spread Method is usually more effective than the Peripheral Glow Method. Both methods permit a continuous self-viewing of the aura which helps the self-intervention effort.

Both the Peripheral Glow and Finger-Spread Methods are valued for their capacity to stimulate and spontaneously unleash our inner psychic powers. When appropriately applied, they can effectively activate our imagery and clairvoyance faculties which are considered essential for viewing the aura and making minor adjustments in its functions during hypnosis. The Finger-Spread Method is more effective in stimulating our PK capacity which is required for direct intervention of the aura's structure, particularly in repairing damage to the aura system. It is very important to note that both methods can be used to achieve highly personal empowerment goals, such as reducing stress, building self-esteem, overcoming growth blockages, and maximizing our inner potentials.

The preliminary considerations are basically the same for both the Peripheral Glow and Finger-Spread Methods. Approximately one hour should be set aside for the typical session during which there must be no interruptions. A quiet, comfortable, and safe setting is required. Minimizing resistance by giving oneself permission to enter the trance state is essential to both procedures. Prior to induction, goals are formulated and stated as positive affirmations. Here are a few examples: *During hypnosis, the aura enveloping my body will become clearly visible to me. My aura is a part of my total being. As I gain insight into the nature of my aura, I will gain insight into the nature of my existence. I am empowered to interact with my aura and intervene into its functions to bring forth positive change. I will be enriched and empowered by this experience.*

The Peripheral Glow Method

The Peripheral Glow Method, as a trance induction and empowerment procedure, uses certain modified components of the familiar Focal-point Procedure for viewing the aura as discussed in Chapter 3. The method requires a shiny, stationary object that is strategically positioned overhead to facilitate a slightly upward gaze. A shiny tack placed on the ceiling is usually effective.

Step 1. Relaxation. Assume a comfortable, reclining position, with your legs uncrossed and your hands resting to your sides. Slow your breathing, and with your eyes closed, mentally scan your body, beginning at your forehead and slowly progressing downward. Pause at tense, stressed areas and let them fully relax. Upon completing the scan, affirm: *I now give myself permission to enter hypnosis. During the trance state, I will be empowered to view my aura and intervene into its functions. I will end the trance state whenever I decide to do so.*

Step 2. Eye Fixation. As you remain relaxed, open your eyes and gaze upward at the shiny object positioned overhead.

Gradually expand your peripheral vision in all directions around the object. Once you reach your peripheral limits, let your eyes go slightly out of focus. You will then notice a white glow enveloping the shiny object. Continue to focus on the object until the glow expands to the limits of your peripheral vision, then close your eyes and let them return to normal. Notice the deep relaxation flooding over your body. To deepen the trance state to the desired level, envision a calm, relaxing scene—a fluffy cloud, a sail in the breeze, or a moon-lit landscape—as you slowly count backward from ten to one.

Step 3. Inner and Outer Body Viewing. The goal of this step is to exercise your ability to mentally view your physical body from both an inner and outer focal point. Your inner view is a function of your internal locus of perception, whereas your outer view is a function of your external locus of perception. To activate your inner viewing capacity, focus on your physical body, passively at rest, from an internal perspective. Notice the physical sensations—warmth, tingling, and so-forth—occurring within and extending to the surface of your body. Following a few moments of sensate-focusing from your inner focal point, extend your perception outwardly beyond your physical body, and note your physical surroundings from your internal locus of perception. Take sufficient time for a detailed picture of your surroundings to emerge. After a brief period of focusing outwardly from your inner perspective, activate your outer viewing capacity by shifting your locus of perception externally and viewing your physical body as though you were an outside observer. From this outside perspective, note the position of your body, and the nature of your clothing. As you form this outer view of your body, make no effort to disengage full consciousness from your physical body. Although a part of your awareness is projected, your inner consciousness must remain securely united with the physical for the duration of this procedure. You can ensure that union by joining the tips of your thumb and middle finger of each hand periodically throughout the procedure while affirming: *I am at complete oneness with* *my total myself—mentally, physically, and spiritually.* This gesture will neither interrupt the trance state nor impair your ability to objectively view and interact with your aura.

Step 4. Remote Aura Viewing. The goal of this stage is to bring your aura into full view from your external locus of perception. To initiate remote aura viewing, objectively focus on your forehead from your external perspective, then gradually expand your peripheral vision to take in the full surroundings of your body. Let your focus shift slightly and you will see a white glow, first around your head and then gradually expanding to envelop your full body. Focus on the white glow as it slowly fades and becomes replaced by the colorful aura. With the aura now visible, notice its coloration, structural characteristics, and other specific features and designs. Pay particular attention to its unique patterns and color characteristics. You are now viewing your aura from your external locus of perception.

Step 5. Aura Interaction and Intervention. As your aura remains visible through remote viewing, use imagery and positive thought messages, both of which are forms of energy, to induce desired changes in the aura's color and energy characteristics. To improve color, first note any area of dullness or deficient coloration. Visualize the desired color and use thought messages to project it to the targeted location in your aura. Once the color infusion process is complete, use additional imagery and appropriate affirmations to blend the color energy into surrounding areas. To enliven the total aura with bright new energy, visualize radiant energy emanating from the aura's core to infuse the visible aura with brilliance. From your external locus of perception, note the expansion of your aura as it absorbs the bright energy. To conclude the interaction process, shift your locus of perception inward by noting your breathing and various physical sensations—warmth, tingling, pressure, weight, and so forth. Sense the peace and serenity permeating your being, along with the powerful balance of your mind, body, and spirit. Audibly affirm: *I am inwardly and outwardly* *balanced. My total being is energized and attuned.* At this point, you can introduce additional personal empowerment goals as you envision them as future realities and affirm your power to achieve them.

Step 6. Trance Exit. With your locus of perception securely centered within yourself, you are now ready to end the trance state by simply stating your intent and then slowly counting from one to five as follows: *I will now come out of hypnosis by counting from one to five. Upon the count of five, I will open my eyes, being fully alert, fully energized, and fully empowered. One, two, three, four, and finally, five.*

Step 7. Resolution. Review the trance experience, paying particular attention to its energizing effects. Sense the vitality of your surrounding energy system, and your inner state of peace, balance, and well-being. Conclude the experience with a few moments of quiet reflection followed by the affirmation, *I am fully empowered mentally, physically, and spiritually.*

The Finger-Spread Method

The Finger-Spread Method, while similar in some ways to the Peripheral Glow Method, is important as a trance induction and aura intervention strategy because of its unique capacity to activate the PK (psychokinesis) faculty. Once activated through this procedure, PK can be used to modify certain dysfunctional aspects of the aura, including fissures, voids, and areas of serious discoloration. Here is the procedure:

Step 1. Mental Passivity. While in a comfortable seated or slightly reclining position, rest your hands, palm sides down, on your thighs, and give yourself permission to fully relax. Let your mind become increasingly passive by intercepting all active thought and deliberately banishing it. Remain in a state of mental passivity for several moments.

Step 2. Trance Induction. To induce the trance state, first focus your attention on your hands, noting each sensation—warmth, coolness, tingling, numbness, moisture in your palms, the texture of your clothing, pressure of your hands against your thighs, and so forth. Next, spread the fingers of either hand and hold the tense, spread position. Then begin slowly relaxing your hand as you affirm: *I now give myself permission to enter hypnosis. By simply relaxing my hand, I will induce the trance state. As my hand relaxes, I am slowly entering hypnosis. Once my hand is fully relaxed, I will be in a deep trance. I will use the trance to view my aura and empower it. I will remain in full control for the duration of the trance experience. I will come out of hypnosis at will.*

Once your hand is fully relaxed, you can deepen the trance state as needed by slowly counting backward from ten, intermittently suggesting deeper relaxation until you reach the desired level.

Step 3. Aura Viewing. The goal of this step is to extend your perceptual capacities beyond your physical body in order to observe your aura. In achieving that goal, it is important to retain your inner sensory awareness while extending your extrasensory awareness. To reach that extended state of awareness, visualize your physical body and objectively observe it. From that external perspective, note the position of your body as it rests peacefully in the trance state. Then focus your attention on your forehead and gradually expand your peripheral vision until a white glow appears around your body. Focus on the transient glow until it is replaced by the colorful aura. With the aura now in view, notice its myriad of features, especially its characteristic coloration, expansiveness, and unique patterns. Give particularly attention to interruptions in energy patterns, including voids, fissures, and discoloration.

Step 4. PK Intervention. With your aura now in view, use the powers of your mind to guide your intervention efforts. Specifically focus your psychic energies on any malfunction in your aura system. Should voids be present, mentally erect a bright dome over the void that slowly fills with radiant energy. For fissures, mentally draw bright strands of energy from the surrounding area and use them as a suture to close the fissure. For areas of discoloration, mentally form a mass of white energy and use it like a sponge to bathe the discolored area and restore brilliance. To infuse the total aura with bright energy, focus on the inner core of your aura system and envision it as a pulsating generator of pure energy, dispersing radiant light in all directions. Mentally observe the infusion process as it occurs throughout your total aura system. At this point, you can specify additional goals, including highly personal ones. Envision them and affirm your determination to achieve them.

Step 5. Conclusion and Resolution. In this final step, the trance state is ended and the empowering effects of the procedure are reviewed. To end the trance, focus your full attention inward and state your intent to exit hypnosis by counting slowly from one to five. On the count of five, open your eyes and take a few moments to reflect on the experience. Note your sense of renewal and vitality. Conclude the procedure with empowering affirmations such as the following: *Every fiber of my being is energized and empowered with positive energy. I am protected and secure. I am at peace within myself. Mentally, physically, and spiritually, I am balanced and attuned to the universe. I am empowered to overcome every obstacle and to achieve my highest goals.*

All the potential benefits of aura intervention by trained specialists are available to us through our own self-intervention strategies. In the end, the ultimate aura specialist resides within yourself. It awaits your recognition, beckons your interaction, and eagerly embraces your empowerment efforts.

7

Aura Power Tools

*Just as our eyes need light in order to see,
our minds need ideas in order to conceive.*

—Nicholas Malebranche,
De la Recherche de la vérité
(1674-75)

A S BIOLOGICAL BEINGS, we exist in a physical world which provides the essential support system and resources for our physical survival—the air we breathe, the food we eat, and the water we drink. Unfortunately, we have recklessly exploited many of the earth's natural resources. We have polluted the air, depleted our forests, and we are rapidly running out of clean, pure water. As a result, our future and that of our children are now at risk. The psychic empowerment perspective emphasizes the importance of responsible action in promoting not only our own personal well being, but that of others and future generations as well.

The temporal dimension in which we now exist is not only essential to our biological survival, it provides an environment for our personal fulfillment and spiritual evolution. Each of its components is a potential empowerment tool. We are inspired by the beauty of the earth's mountains, rivers, oceans, and plains. The primeval forest with its towering trees, lush undergrowth, and verdant floor energizes us with a deeper awareness of the infinite power behind all creation. The earth's majestic mountains challenge us not only to scale their heights, but more importantly, to reach our own peaks of awareness and power. The unparalleled force of the ever expanding universe with its billions of galaxies, some of them intersecting to spin off new galaxies, reminds us of the selfsame force that underlies and sustains our own existence.

We can scarcely comprehend the scope and splendor of creation and the infinite force behind it; yet the magnificence of the cosmos parallels in many ways the beauty and masterful design of our own existence. The energizing hub of the cosmos, for instance, is the compeer of the energizing inner core of our own being. Moreover, we, like the cosmos, are constantly evolving. Wondrous growth resources with inexhaustible possibilities exist both within ourselves and throughout the universe. We are endowed with limitless empowerment potential and surrounded by an endless array of empowerment tools. A major focus of the psychic empowerment perspective is the discovery of tangible tools with capacities to empower our lives, and the development of strategies that effectively apply them. Through appropriate power tools and strategies, we can unleash the infinite power underlying the cosmos and our own existence.

The tangible tools of psychic empowerment are infinite in both number and variation. They can range from a simple object that holds special meaning to a distant star that commands our attention and gives us new hope. They can be as simple as a bird in flight, a leaf carried by the wind, or a mystical moonlit cove. They can be certain places we go for renewal and inspiration. They can consist of a snow-covered landscape, an exciting summer rainstorm, or a beautiful sunset—each with power to lift awareness and energize our lives.

Experiences with our natural surroundings during our developmental years can be particularly empowering. A college professor remembered a rock ledge overlooking an emerald-green lake as personally empowering to him during his teen years. "Its beauty and serenity," he recalled, "drew me back to it time and time again. The tranquil scene became so etched in my mind that I still call it forth as a source of inspiration and power." A nurse recalled a giant oak under which she often played as a child as especially empowering to her. "Its checkered shade is still a carefree playground in my mind."

Many tangibles are empowering primarily because of their associative value. Among the familiar examples are heirlooms or objects that came to us as gifts. A professional athlete recalls, "For me, a high school graduation gift of a fountain pen from my father held special significance. As a college student, I discovered that writing with this special pen seemed to stimulate my thinking and unleash the flow of new ideas. The 'magic pen' became an important empowerment tool throughout my college years."

Because of the interactive nature of our existence, any condition or experience that is empowering to us mentally, physically, or spiritually is likewise empowering to the aura system. Profound experiences, such as the peak experience and the so-called "ah ha!" experience, not only enlighten us mentally, they also illuminate and revitalize the aura. Similarly, meaningful interactions with nature and the insight we gain through nature's harbingers are often permanently empowering to our total being. This was illustrated by a college student who found solace in a bright shooting star that streaked across the summer sky shortly after her brother's sudden death in an auto crash. She saw the shooting star as a signal of her brother's joyful transition to a beautiful dimension of light and love. The experience lasted only seconds, but its empowering effects were enduring. In a similar instance, a college administrator, despondent over a diagnosis of a life-threatening illness, discovered a totally new dimension to her life when an aged magnolia tree, visible from her office window, unexpectedly burst forth in full bloom, flooding her office with its fresh, energizing fragrance. The magical experience was a turning point in her life. Inspired and empowered, she entered the most productive and rewarding phase of her life. Now fully recovered from an illness which had seemed at first a death sentence, she asserts with great confidence, "I was resurrected by an aged magnolia tree."

The Empowerment Nature Walk

Many of us have already discovered that our spontaneous interactions with the earth can be enormously empowering. A leisurely stroll on the beach or walk in the forest is often enough to clear the mind, revitalize the body, and literally illuminate the aura. The rich benefits of these spontaneous interactions suggest the possibility that structured strategies could be equally or perhaps even more effective in empowering our lives. The Empowerment Nature Walk is a structured procedure designed to energize the aura and, at the same time, empower us to achieve specifically designated personal goals through guided interactions with nature.

Anyone can benefit from the Empowerment Nature Walk. It can generate insight, solve problems, stimulate creativity, reduce stress, promote wellness, and unleash the flow of vibrant energy. Individuals who have lost hope or who are encountering reversals in either their personal life or career often find invaluable new resources through this procedure. The rewards of the walk are immediate and usually lasting.

Although most natural settings are appropriate for the Empowerment Nature Walk, a scenic vista with a winding trail or an old-growth forest with its community of life provides the ideal condition. Simply touching a magnificent tree or breathing in the fragrance of a flower can brighten the aura. Here is the procedure:

Step 1. Aura Preview. Before starting the walk, view your aura using any of the self-viewing techniques previously discussed.

Step 2. Goal Statement. Settle back and with your eyes closed, formulate your immediate goals and state them as specifically as possible. Ask yourself, "What do I hope to accomplish through this walk in nature?" Your goal may be simply to energize your aura system or to experience the sheer pleasure of the walk. On the other hand, you may want to overcome a certain growth blockage in your life, gain insight into yourself, find a solution to a particular problem, or resolve a personal conflict.

Step 3. The Walk. Select a safe, familiar place for walking. Walk at a comfortable pace, taking time to notice your surroundings. Think of the elements around you—plants, animals, rocks, and streams—as energized creations of nature with power to share. Let them speak to you as you absorb the vibrant energy gathering around you. Think of your surroundings as partners in your empowerment journey. Enjoy the miracles of life around you. Note your sense of oneness with nature, and tell yourself, *I am an integral part of all that exists.* Review your goals as formulated in Step 1, and affirm your power to achieve them.

Step 4. Reflection. At the end of the walk, look back on the experience and reflect on the interactions that occurred. Formulate detailed mental images related to the walk and file them away as snapshots in your mind for future reference. Review the empowering effects of the walk, then affirm: *I am empowered by this experience. By calling forth images related to it, I can at any moment unleash the flow of vibrant energy in my life.*

Step 5. Aura Post-view and Evaluation. View your aura again, using the same self-viewing technique as in Step 1, and note the changes. Re-affirm the empowering effects of the experience.

The Empowerment Nature Walk, although relatively structured, is sufficiently flexible that it can be practiced under wide-ranging conditions. It can include night and day walks, as well as walks with a partner or animal pets. Walks by moonlight are especially empowering. Group walks are also highly effective, particularly when they include follow-up discussions of the experience.

The Empowerment Nature Walk can be adapted to a variety of age groups ranging from preschoolers to the aged. It can increase our awareness of our natural surroundings and help us to discover the value of our interactions with nature. The procedure can be easily integrated into a variety of instructional programs, particularly courses involving the appreciation and preservation of our natural resources.

The Empowerment Nature Walk is a particularly useful strategy for releasing tension and generating a sense of well-being. Peaceful serenity almost invariably accompanies the experience, and spontaneous solutions to problems often emerge during the walk. This was illustrated by an engineer who used the procedure to resolve an important career issue. He recalls, "A few years ago, I was faced with the dilemma of choosing between two career options, each with advantages and disadvantages. My analysis of the situation only confused me further. During a late afternoon walk along a nature trail, the solution spontaneously came to me. I chose the option revealed by the walk, and my career flourished. To have gone with the other option would have put my career on hold."

The Empowerment Nature Walk typically includes multiple interactions with many objects of nature. The result is usually a generalized state of empowerment along with specialized benefits related to particular goals. The long term effects of the procedure can be reinforced by periodically evoking any of the images related to the experience.

The effectiveness of the Empowerment Nature Walk suggests that other more focused procedures designed to provide interactions with specifically designated natural objects would likewise be empowering. The tree, moon, and stars are among nature's tangibles with immense empowerment potential when incorporated as power tools into structured procedures.

Tree Power Interaction

Tree Power Interaction is a structured, specialized procedure that utilizes the tree as a tangible, interactive object. It recognizes our natural tendency to interact with nature, and the empowerment possibilities of those interactions. More specifically, it emphasizes the enormously empowering potential of our interactions with various trees, and the differential effects of those interactions on the aura system.

The tree is a complex energy system which continues to grow throughout its lifetime. Some trees, among them the giant redwoods, have stood for more than 3,000 years. As the planet's oldest and largest living thing, the towering tree is the earth's antenna to the universe. It is a tangible reminder of our own connection to the cosmos and our capacity for endless growth.

Although all trees can be seen as generators of energy, the empowering influences of trees vary, depending on the characteristics of the tree and the nature of our interactions with it. Typically, the older the tree the more inspiring and energizing its effects. The seasons of the year do not appear to influence the tree's empowerment significance.

Tree Power Interaction as an aura empowerment exercise requires specific goals and the selection of an appropriate tree. The tree is seen as a cooperative partner rather than merely a tangible object to be used as an empowerment tool for gaining a particular goal. Awareness of the tree as a power system, and recognition of its splendor as a masterful creation of nature are critical to the success of the procedure.

In Tree Power Interaction, the tree selection process initiates the empowerment interaction. We select the tree, but at the same time, the tree selects us. This interaction is particularly evident among trees that attract our attention and inspire us by their stateliness and beauty. Some trees seem to literally call out to us as though they recognize our empowerment needs. They quietly compel us to touch them, interact with them, and draw power from them. Here are a few examples of the differential effects of various trees on the human aura:

The Regal Oak

This is both an all-purpose tree and an all-time favorite. In our survey of 350 students selected randomly from a college population, over eighty percent identified the oak as their favorite tree. Such a strong preference could be largely due to the spontaneously energizing effects of the mighty oak on the human energy system. The sheer presence of the oak expands the aura while banishing discoloration and introducing a variety of bright colors. By deliberately interacting with this stately tree, we can further illuminate the aura and expand its boundaries to accommodate an even wider range of new color energies, depending on our empowerment goals.

The Amiable Poplar

The poplar was ranked second in our survey of college students as the tree they preferred most. Healing and rejuvenating energies seem to emanate from this amiable tree. Its energy frequencies are finely tuned, and they tend to attune and balance the human aura system. Visual inspection of the aura during physical contact with the poplar typically reveals a stabilizing effect along with certain color changes, including a bright infusion of light rose at the visible aura's outer edge.

Photographs of the poplar leaf using electrophotographic procedures show an intricate, symmetrical pattern of expansive energy surrounding the leaf. The *phantom leaf effect,* a relatively rare phenomenon in which the energy pattern enveloping a full leaf remains intact even after a part of the leaf is removed, typically characterizes the poplar leaf. This phenomenon reflects the tree's physical restoration tendencies and the healing power of its abundant energy system. Any physical exposure to the poplar is health enhancing.

Although the health claims associated with this tree may seem to some more like magic than science, there is considerable research evidence that Tree Power Interaction using the poplar tree can promote physical health. Our laboratory studies found that the aura often becomes discolored and unbalanced immediately prior to the onset of physical illness. Interaction with the poplar tree infuses the aura with bright, healthful energy, an effect which is visible throughout the aura immediately following the interaction.

It would follow that multiple interactions with the poplar tree could effectively build our resistance to disease, a conclusion that is supported by at least two studies. College students who practiced Tree Power Interaction with the poplar at frequent intervals during a cold and flu season reported fewer instances of illness when compared to a control group that did not practice the procedure. In another study investigating the health effects of the procedure, subjects with a history of recurring tension headaches experienced a progressive decline in both frequency and intensity of their headaches, effects they attributed to their daily interactions with the poplar tree.

Aside from its physical health benefits, Tree Power Interaction with the poplar has shown considerable promise as a mental health strategy. In our studies, patients experiencing depression or anxiety found that even limited interactions with this tree increased their feelings of self-worth and gave them new hope. The procedure was found to be particularly effective in reducing anxiety and fear associated with panic disorders and phobias. Also, patients experiencing insomnia found they fell asleep faster, and their sleep was less disturbed following their interactions with the poplar. Our studies found that a leaf taken from the tree and placed under the pillow in an envelope further promoted the empowering effects of this procedure. Almost without exception, guided practice using this procedure gave our subjects a sense of power over their symptoms and increased their belief in themselves.

Although more research is needed to assess the physical and mental health benefits of this strategy, present findings suggest that almost everyone can benefit from interactions with this amicable tree.

The Vigorous Pine

Interactions with the pine tree tend to generate an abundant but often transient supply of powerful energy which is usually visible as increased brilliance in the aura. Many real-life situations require an immediate, forceful surge of new energy. Common examples are the many stressful conditions of daily life, including career and family-related demands, that can deplete our energy supply. Pine tree interactions revitalize the aura, often with visible flashes of new energy, including red which seems to jump-start the aura's energizing capacities. The result is a total infusion of abundant energy.

Interactions with the pine are particularly valuable in helping us remain controlled and poised under pressure. In our research, managers who practiced Tree Power Interaction with the pine reported a marked improvement in their management skills, particularly in working with difficult people.

The Stalwart Hickory

Interactions with this tree are associated with positive social relationships, personal achievement, accelerated learning, and emotional stability. The resultant changes in the aura system typically include a bright infusion of yellow, particularly to the aura's inner regions. Individuals who are undergoing transition in their personal lives or careers are particularly energized by interactions with this tree.

The cognitive effects of interacting with the hickory include both accelerated learning and better retention. Our studies found that college students who had been placed on academic probation rapidly improved in their coursework, and eventually, they raised their overall grade-point averages through regular interactions with the hickory tree. Moreover, the rewards associated with this tree were found to be long lasting.

The Perpetual Cedar

The cedar is a powerful tree that symbolizes permanence and endurance. It withstands the elements and the ravishes of time. Interactions with this rugged tree fortify the aura with an abundant energy supply that resists any intrusion of external forces, including those that could otherwise drain our energy system. When the aura system is under attack, interactions with the cedar tree provide an outer shield of protection which envelops the total aura. Areas of aura weakness and vulnerability, such as voids and fissures, usually remain evident, but they become securely enclosed within the protective shield.

Other tree interactions include the walnut which introduces brown into the aura and is associated with practicality; the beech which introduces orange and is associated with financial success; the redwood which, like the cedar, reinforces the aura and is associated with permanence and endurance; the sycamore which expands the aura and is associated with self-discovery and insight; the spruce and fir, both of which energize the aura, are associated with achievement; and the ginkgo which introduces purple and is associated with psychic development and universal wisdom. The degree of change in the aura usually depends on the intensity and frequency of our interactions with the tree.

Tree Power Interaction requires the physical presence of a tree as the empowerment object. Critical to the success of the procedure are clear empowerment goals and the selection of a tree appropriate to those goals. The procedure begins and ends with aura viewings which provide a basis for evaluating the effectiveness of the procedure. Here is the procedure:

Step 1. Aura Viewing. View your aura, using any of the self-viewing procedures previously discussed. Note particularly the color, brightness, and magnitude of your aura.

Step 2. Goal Statement. Formulate your goal(s) for the interaction. Your goal may be to infuse your aura with healthful energy, energize a dormant region in your energy system, add color to the aura, correct an energy dysfunction, or illuminate the total aura, to list but a few of the possibilities. Other goals not directly related to the aura can involve an unlimited range of personal concerns, including physical, emotional, social, career, and so forth.

Step 3. Tree Selection. Selecting a tree initiates the interactive process. It is important to select a tree that appeals to you personally and seems appropriate for your particular goals. It can be a familiar tree or one that you notice for the first time. It can be either isolated or closely surrounded by other trees. Once you select a tree, note your sense of connection to it. Before approaching the tree, interact with it by observing its unique characteristics such as height, proportions, and structure. Mentally engage the tree as a receptive partner in your empowerment efforts. Acknowledge the tree as a magnificent creation of nature with an abundant supply of energy.

Step 4. Tree Power Infusion. As you approach the tree, sense its surrounding field of energy interacting with your own energy field. Touch the tree first with your fingertips, thereby connecting the antennae of your body to the tree as the powerful antenna of the earth. Note the wondrous infusion of cosmic energy permeating your total energy system. Rest your palms against the tree and note an even greater infusion of intense power. Your total being is now linked not only to the tree, but to the limitless power of the cosmos.

Step 5. Tree Power Interaction. With your palms resting against the tree, visualize your aura system interacting with the energy system of the tree. Sense the powerful changes occurring in your aura system, from its outer edges to its innermost core. Gently stroke the tree, and let the tree speak to you. Reaffirm your connection to the infinite power of the cosmos.

Step 6. Reflection. Disengage the tree and bring your hands together in a praying hands position. Reflect on the powerful interaction experience. Look upward at the tree as you review your empowerment goals. Address the tree and affirm your goals as present realities. For instance, if your goal is to energize your aura, affirm: *I am totally infused mentally, physically, and spiritually with abundant energy,* as you envision your aura glowing with bright energy. If your goal is better health, affirm: *I am now fully infused with healthful energy.* If your goal is to quit smoking, affirm: *I am now smoke-free.* Even goals concerning the distant future can be stated as present realities. If you are a student and your goal is future career success, affirm: *Career success is my destiny.* Accompany your affirmations with goal-related imagery to further strengthen the empowering effects of the procedure.

Step 7. Aura post-view and Evaluation. View your aura and compare it to your earlier viewing. Note the changes, particular in coloration, brightness, and magnitude.

Following the procedure, periodically reflecting on the experience as images of the tree are formed can instantly reactivate the procedure's empowerment results.

Almost everyone who practices Tree Power Interaction develops an empowerment affiliation with certain trees that hold special meanings for them personally. Among my favorite trees for this exercise is an enormous oak standing on the grounds in front of my office. A century-old majestic work of nature, it seems to disperse empowering energy in all directions. A few years ago, it was struck by lightening but miraculously withstood the assault, which left only a character scar down its rugged trunk. Today, it remains a regal model of immense power, symmetrically poised to interact with all who come near it.

The Moon Power Strategy

The moon, our only natural satellite and nearest neighbor in space, has steadfastly inspired poets, authors, musicians, scientists, and artists for centuries. Shakespeare likened it to "a silver bow newbent in heaven." Shelley described it as "that orbed maiden, with white fire laden, whom mortals call the moon." Musicians, inspired by the moon, wrote such popular songs as *Blue Moon, Moonlight and Roses, Moonlight Bay, Moon Over Miami, Moon River, By the Light of the Silvery Moon,* and *Shine On, Harvest Moon. Moonlight Sonata* is one of Beethoven's most beloved works.

Many early civilizations attributed god-like qualities to the moon. The ancient Romans called their moon Diana, goddess of the hunt, whose bow was the crescent moon and whose arrows were moonbeams. Native Americans, along with many other civilizations, measured time by the moon. "Many moons ago" and "once in a blue moon" are contemporary remnants of that tradition.

Speculations abound concerning the moon and its powers. The moon is known, of course, to cause tides, and research has suggested that it can assert a direct influence on human behavior. We have already alluded to the moon's inspirational effects as reflected in the many magnificent creations of civilizations past and present. Like the ancients, we are still enchanted by the moon's beauty and mystery. It captures our imagination and stimulates our artistic expression, while contributing a rich, magical dimension to our existence.

The spontaneous power of the moon to inspire the noblest expressions of the human mind suggests many important empowerment possibilities. In hypnosis, for instance, simple imagery of the moon can increase receptivity to the induction procedure. Hypnosis subjects often report that the very sound of the word moon induces a serene mental state and increases responsiveness to suggestion. As a post-hypnotic cue, imagery of the moon is one of the most powerful tools known for activating the empowerment potential of suggestions presented during hypnosis.

Our early efforts to develop empowerment strategies related to the moon suggested that either viewing the full moon, or merely envisioning it, tended to illuminate and expand the aura. We later found that a sphere of new color and the energies related to it could be introduced into the aura by simply envisioning a moon of the desired color. We then discovered that the sphere of color energy could be deliberately targeted to a designated area within the aura where it could either remain in concentrated energy form, or be dispersed throughout the aura system. For instance, green as a healing color could be introduced to envelop the aura system with a healthful shield, or it could be guided as a concentrated sphere to a specific dysfunctional region where it remained in undiluted form until the repair mission was accomplished. Other spheres of energy could be introduced to infuse the aura with a new region or layer of color, with the placement of the sphere in the aura usually related to the color's empowerment significance. For example, yellow as a cognitive growth color is usually introduced in concentrated form in the aura's uppermost region, whereas pink as a rejuvenating color is usually introduced as an inner layer of youthful energy that fully envelops the physical body.

Following several pilot studies, we developed the Moon Power Strategy which utilizes the full moon as a tangible tool, or when the moon is absent, imagery of the moon, to introduce empowering change into the aura system. Here is the strategy:

Step 1. Initial Aura Viewing. View your aura using any of the full-aura viewing techniques previously discussed. Pay particular attention to the aura's coloration and intervention needs.

Step 2. Goal Formulation. Specifically state your aura intervention goals, and then affirm: *I will use this procedure to achieve these goals.*

Step 3. Moon Viewing. View the full moon, or when the moon is absent, form a mental picture of it. Allow the image of the moon to become firmly fixed in your mind.

Step 4. Moon Imagery. With your eyes closed, envision the full moon and focus your full attention on it. Exclude all other images from your mind. Allow sufficient time for the moon to vividly appear.

Step 5. Empowerment Activity. With the full moon image firmly fixed in your mind, recall each of your goals and engage the moon as your empowerment partner. If your goal is to infuse your aura with brightness, envision the moon as radiating bright energy and your total aura system absorbing it. If your goal is to add a particular color to a designated area in your aura, envision the moon taking on that color and transferring it either as moon beams or as a sphere of color to your aura, infusing the designated area with new energy. If your goal is to introduce a new rim of color into your aura, envision the moon changing to that color and dispersing it as bright energy to your full aura.

Step 6. Final Aura Viewing. View your aura again, using the same viewing procedure as in Step 1. Note the changes in your aura. Conclude the exercise with the simple affirmation: *I am fully empowered.*

The long-term results of the Moon Power Strategy depend on several influencing factors. Among the most critical are the nature of your empowerment needs and the intensity of the energy concentration introduced into your aura. For some needs, a single intervention effort is sufficient, but for others, repeat interventions are required. A void in the aura or an area of discoloration typically requires a single intervention; whereas serious structural damage to the aura may require numerous sessions. As a general rule, a new color introduced into the aura is somewhat transient. Frequent interventions over time are required for such long-range goals as rejuvenation and physical fitness.

The Star Power Strategy

Deep within each of us is the aura's innermost core of energy, the centerpoint of power that energies our being. It can be thought of as the inner life force which is the sum and substance of our existence as a conscious entity in the universe. Its perpetual nature assures our continuation beyond physical life and from life to life. It is our contact with the infinite power of the cosmos. When we are attuned to the core of energy within, and to the higher source of power in the cosmos, we experience the ultimate state of cosmic attunement, a phenomenon also known as cosmic congruency.

We have all experienced instances of spontaneous cosmic attunement. Examples are our many interactions with nature that lift awareness to new levels, and those rich moments of joy, love, and peace that we all experience from day to day. The frequency of these experiences reflects our innate potential for cosmic attunement on a larger scale.

The Star Power Strategy is a structured procedure designed to generate a state of complete cosmic attunement. The procedure is similar to the Cosmic Centering Procedure as previously discussed in that it attempts to re-connect and attune us to the cosmos. It is unique, however, in that it introduces a star as our link to the cosmic dimension of our existence.

The Star Power Strategy grew out of an experiment in which forty-five students enrolled in an evening parapsychology course at Athens State University were given six sequential tasks. They were first instructed to envision the distant side of the universe and describe what they saw. They experienced considerable difficulty completing this task, with most of them eventually reporting only darkness or nothing at all. The group was then instructed to envision the energy core of the universe and describe what they saw. They were unusually successful in completing this task with thirty-one of the forty-five students reporting either brightness or a bright life force.

The group of students were then escorted outside the classroom and instructed to select a star and while viewing it, imagine it to be a miniature replica of the giant core of the cosmos. They were then instructed to close their eyes, form an image of the star they had just viewed, and as before, imagine it as a replica of the core of the cosmos. Without exception, they reported success in completing this task. They were then instructed to envision a beam of light connecting the star to the brilliant hub of the cosmos. Once again, they were all successful at this task. Finally, they were instructed to envision a beam of light connecting them to the star and indirectly to the bright core of the cosmos. They were all successful in completing this task, including the fourteen students who had previously experienced difficulty envisioning the energy core of the universe.

Based on the findings of this exercise, we developed the Star Power Strategy utilizing either a visible star or an image of it as the empowerment object. Instead of viewing the aura, this procedure requires scanning the aura, a mental exercise designed to sense the aura and its frequency patterns. Here is the procedure:

Step 1. Body Scan. Settle back, take in a few deep breaths, and let your mind become passive by clearing it of active thought. With your mind emptied of problems, mentally scan your physical body, beginning at the upper region and progressing slowly downward. Note any build-up of tension and mentally release it.

Step 2. Aura Scan. This step requires three mental scans of the aura—the energy scan, color scan, and structural scan. With your eyes closed, envision the full aura enveloping your physical body. Then, beginning above your head, slowly scan your aura downward as you sense its energy frequencies. Note any disruption or interference in energy patterns. Having completed the energy scan, conduct a color scan, again beginning at the aura's uppermost region and progressing slowly downward. Allow images of the aura's color make-up to accompany the scan, including regions and enveloping layers of color as well as areas of discoloration. Finally, conduct a structural scan of the aura beginning again at the aura's uppermost region. Note particular structural features, paying special attention to possible dysfunctions, such as voids, breaks, or fissures.

Step 3. Star View. Scan the night sky and select a certain star for viewing. If a star is not visible, form a mental image of one. Focus your full attention on the star, whether real or imagined, and sense your personal connection to it. Give the star a name—any name that comes to mind—and address the star as your intimate link to the cosmos. Think of it as a miniature but powerful replica of the cosmic core. Imagine the star connected to the center of the cosmos by a beam of light and endowed with the same limitless power as the cosmic core.

Step 4. Power Draw. Envision your aura and a beam of light connecting it to the star. Visualize bright cosmic energy from the star progressively infusing your aura system, beginning at your aura's upper region and gradually moving downward. Sense the pulsating energy as it fills your aura, infusing voids and repairing dysfunctional or damaged regions. Sense the harmonious vibrations within your aura as it becomes filled with vibrant cosmic energy.

Step 5. Final Aura Scan. As you sense pulsating cosmic energy infusing your aura system, mentally scan your aura from its upper region downward. Note its vibrancy, balance, and attunement. Sense harmonious frequencies throughout your aura system. You are now attuned to the innermost core of your being and to the powerful core of the cosmos.

Step 6. Conclusion. Conclude the exercise with the simple assertion: *My total being is infused and empowered with pure cosmic energy.*

Up until now, our discussion of empowerment tangibles has focused on our natural surroundings and the larger system of the universe. The earth, moon, stars, and the distant reaches of the cosmos are constant reminders of the power of creation. They invite our interaction and challenge our probes. They are accessible at any time, and their resources are inexhaustible.

Also available to us are many other empowerment tangibles of lesser magnitude but of equal significance. They range from highly personalized objects that, over time, assume important empowerment properties to the many concrete objects which are valued on a broader, often cultural scale for their empowerment relevance.

The empowering effects of tangible objects can be explained from several perspectives. One view holds that certain objects are actively empowering because of their intrinsic nature. Common examples are the quartz crystal, the pyramid, and various gems. Some of these objects are thought to be energizing by their sheer presence, independent of our interactions or associations with them. Others are believed to require our active participation in order to access their empowering properties.

Many tangible objects are considered inert yet potentially empowering because of their psychological significance. They assume psychological importance only when we ascribe certain empowering properties to them. Examples are the use of certain tangible objects as post-hypnotic cues to activate hypnotic suggestions, and the placebo or expectancy effects of certain objects, such as a good-luck charm or a special article of clothing. The empowerment results are due to the associations we form with these objects rather than the intrinsic nature of the object itself.

Certain objects are considered empowering because of their capacity to link us to important new sources of knowledge. They serve primarily as information channels. Examples are the pendulum, dowsing rods, and table tilting. Physical contact with these objects is usually required to initiate their retrieval capacities. The information acquired through these objects emanates either from an outside power source or from the handler's subconscious rather than from the object. These objects, consequently, are considered inert and powerless except for their capacity to access other power sources.

Many tangible objects are empowering primarily because of their culturally ascribed significance. Examples in our culture are money, stocks and bonds, awards, diplomas, and a variety of concrete status symbols. Unfortunately, certain of these tangibles, while potentially empowering, can assume disempowering properties. Money, for instance, is almost always associated with power and status, but when it becomes a controlling force in our lives, the end result can be tragedy. Familiar examples are the suicides often attributed to the loss of wealth.

Certain objects are empowering because of their symbolic significance. They can inspire dedication, service, and sacrifice. A common example is the national flag as a symbol of freedom and patriotism. We pledge allegiance to it and in song, we personify it as gallant and proud. Religions around the world incorporate tangible objects into their rituals to represent commitment, sacrifice, devotion, and in many instances, a divine presence. Examples are the icon, cross, prayer carpet, and shrine.

Because of their unique design and functions, certain tangible objects have particular relevance as aura empowerment tools. Although many of these objects seem to empower the aura by their physical presence, others require strategies that deliberately access their empowerment properties. Some of these tangibles appear to have a single empowering function whereas others seem to possess multiple empowerment properties.

In the discussion that follows, we will explore the relevance of several empowerment tangibles and develop strategies designed to maximize their empowerment capacities. We will focus specifically on the pyramid, quartz crystal, and various precious and semi-precious gems. The pyramid and quartz crystal are often considered all-purposeful as empowerment tools, whereas gems are typically considered more specialized in their empowerment properties. As a general rule, the physical size of the object does not appear to influence its empowerment potential. When appropriately used, a miniature replica of the Great Pyramid, for instance, can be equally as empowering as the Great Pyramid itself. Similarly, a small quartz crystal can be equally as empowering as a larger one. Although our focus here is on the direct relevance of these tools to the human aura, we will at times consider certain other empowerment applications, each of which is at least indirectly related to the aura.

The Pyramid

The pyramid as a tool for psychic empowerment is usually a miniature replica of the Great Pyramid erected by King Khufu near Cairo, Egypt in the 2600s B.C. As already noted, the size of the pyramid does not appear to influence its empowerment properties, nor does its solidity or the materials used in its construction. In our research, we have used pyramids of paper, glass, crystal, wood, metal, amber, marble, alabaster, and plastic, all with apparent equal effectiveness. Although one side of the pyramid is usually aligned to the compass for training purposes, experienced subjects usually find that orienting the pyramid to the compass is not critical to its usefulness as an empowerment tool.

The effectiveness of the pyramid as an empowerment tool remains a mystery. One view holds that the power of the pyramid depends solely on the expectancy effect. From this perspective, the energies we invest in the object and the results we expect from it determine its empowerment effects. This view emphasizes the importance of procedures that emphasize expected outcomes. Within this context, the pyramid is valuable in that it provides a tangible mooring for our expectations, thereby providing them with a dimension of empowering substance.

Another perspective views the pyramid alone as a tool endowed with power rather than simply an inert device or useful means to an end. This view, often labeled pyramid power, holds that the mere presence of the pyramid, even when we are unaware of it, is potentially empowering. The pyramid is seen as either generating empowering energy or else transmitting it from another source. Either way, the pyramid is considered independently empowering in and of itself. This perspective recognizes, however, that our active involvement with the pyramid can significantly increase its empowerment effectiveness.

There is considerable evidence to support the pyramid power view. Our studies found that sales dramatically increased when a small pyramid was concealed in a box over the entrance to a sporting goods business. Similar results were noted for a gift shop and a video rental business. In yet another instance, the founder of an engineering firm known for its phenomenal growth acknowledged that he had strategically position a solid metal pyramid in the concrete foundation of the company's central office building during its construction. He commented, "I was not exactly a believer, but I thought, 'What is there to lose?'" Today, he privately attributes the success of the multi-million dollar business, in great part, to the pyramid. Along a different line, a psychologist found that a small, crystal pyramid concealed under a table at the center of the room in group therapy invariably increased participation and positive group interactions.

Much of our research concerning the pyramid involved its effects on various mental functions, particularly learning and memory. Our studies of college students found that the rate of associative learning of nonsense syllables rapidly increased when a small pyramid of glass was introduced into the learning situation. Furthermore, both short-term and long-term memory improved when the pyramid was present. Even when the pyramid's presence was unknown to the research subjects, significant improvements in both learning and memory were noted. However, even greater improvements were noted when the subjects were informed that a pyramid was present. The most favorable results were obtained when the subjects were informed not only of the pyramid's presence but of its expected empowerment effects as well.

Many of our research subjects, having participated in our pyramid studies, began using the pyramid in their daily lives. Several of them used the pyramid as a study aid throughout their undergraduate and graduate programs. A chemistry major found that a small pyramid of glass either held in his hand or placed on his desk during course exams stimulated his recall of essential course materials. One of our subjects, now a clinical psychologist in private practice, adopted a small quartz pyramid as her "learned partner." She reports, "The pyramid saw me through my doctoral program and is now my 'co-therapist.'" She regularly uses the pyramid as a meditation and hypnosis induction aid. Another research subject, now a practicing attorney, reports that a miniature crystal pyramid, which he continues to carry in his pocket, rescued him from probationary status as an undergraduate political science major and initiated an achievement spiral that saw him through law school and into a successful practice.

Along a different line, there is strong evidence to suggest that the pyramid can be used as a creativity tool. Although creativity has no limits, our access to it can become blocked. The pyramid can unblock our creative potentials and stimulate creative expression. This was illustrated by an art student who, believing he had exhausted his creative capacities, used a crystal pyramid to generate exciting new ideas for his paintings. He applied the pyramid as a point of focus to induce a meditative state, during which he envisioned a large pyramid upon which appeared images of his next painting.

Recent studies suggest numerous applications of the pyramid as a possible health and fitness tool. Our studies found that simply envisioning the pyramid, independent of its physical presence, tends to induce a tranquil, healthy state of mind. Furthermore, there is strong evidence to suggest that the sheer presence of the pyramid can accelerate the healing process. When structured procedures are applied, the health and fitness applications of this tool seem almost unlimited. Examples include managing weight, becoming smoke free, building resistance to illness, and overcoming a host of stress-related disorders. (See *Psychic Empowerment for Health and Fitness* for a detailed description of these applications.)

The Pyramid of Power

The pyramid has particular relevance to our study of the human aura in several ways. Our early investigations of this tool found that simply holding the hands over a pyramid energizes and expands the aura. With the introduction of appropriate imagery, we noted a significant increase in the pyramid's empowering effects. Based on these observations, we developed the Pyramid of Power, a procedure specifically designed to energize, expand, and empower the total aura system. The pyramid model used for this procedure can be of any desired size or material.

Step 1. Preparation and Orientation. Position the pyramid at a comfortable viewing level with one side of the pyramid facing you. As you center your attention on the pyramid, clear your mind and let your body become relaxed. Give yourself permission to become energized through the use of the pyramid as an empowerment tool.

Step 2. Cosmic Connection. Envision a powerful shaft of energy connecting the pyramid's apex to the ultimate source of power—the core of the cosmos. Envision the pyramid, charged with bright cosmic power, radiating pure energy in all directions.

Step 3. Energy Transfer. Hold your hands at opposite sides of the pyramid, with your palms turned toward the pyramid as your contact to the cosmic source of power. Without touching the pyramid, sense its warm, vibrant power resonating in your palms and spreading bright new energy throughout your physical body.

Step 4. Inner Core Infusion. Focus on your solar plexus and its inner core of energy. Visualize the inner core of your being as it becomes infused with power from the pyramid.

Step 5. Aura Infusion. Sense the vibrant energy emanating from your inner core of energy and radiating throughout your aura to permeate your total being with new power. Visualize your aura expanding and glowing with bright energy.

Step 6. Imagery Review. Allow the powerful energy infusion to continue as you review the procedure's empowering sequence:

(A) Envision again powerful cosmic energy entering the pyramid through its apex.

(B) Envision the pyramid, infused with cosmic power, radiating pure energy in all directions.

(C) Sense the energy from the pyramid entering the palms of your hands and subsequently, being transmitted to your energy system's innermost core.

(D) Sense your energy core radiating powerful energy throughout your aura system.

Step 7. Affirmation. Bring your palms together in a praying hands position and with your eyes closed, affirm: *Mentally, physically, and spiritually, I am balanced and attuned to the universe. I am fully infused with bright, positive energy. I am empowered!*

This exercise can be readily adapted to groups, with the pyramid typically positioned on a table at the center of the group. The procedure can also be modified to add color to the aura or to focus on specific deficiencies in the aura. To add a particular color to the aura, envision energy of the desired color being emitted by the pyramid and transferred through the palms to the aura system, or to a targeted area in the aura. To empower a particular region of the aura, such as an area of deficient energy, mentally direct bright energy from your inner core of energy to the designated area.

For health and fitness goals, the procedure can target healing cosmic energy transmitted by the pyramid to specific organs or body regions. A combination of positive affirmation and imagery of healing energy as a ray of light from the pyramid being focused on the target area can effectively accelerate healing as well as control pain. To bathe the aura with luminosity, which is critical to all health and fitness applications, the energy frequencies emitted by the pyramid and concentrated in the aura's inner core are allowed to spread profusely throughout the body, permeating its multiple organs and systems with new vitality and power.

The Pyramid of Power, when practiced regularly, has been effective in spontaneously slowing and arresting the aging process. In instances of premature aging associated with either stress or illness, the procedure can virtually reverse aging. This application was illustrated by a chronic pain patient who practiced the procedure to manage back pain. She promptly took command of the pain, and almost immediately the signs of premature aging began to disappear as her aura assumed a healthy glow.

The Pyramid of Power can have important therapeutic benefits, as illustrated by a sales manager who used the procedure to overcome his fear of flying. Following a single practice sessions, he placed a small crystal pyramid in his pocket and took a cross-country flight with absolutely no fear. "For the first time in my life," he recalls, "I actually enjoyed flying." Now free of the phobia, he flies regularly, but always accompanied by a small pyramid which he calls his "life support system."

In our studies, children with attention deficit/hyperactivity disorders experienced dramatic improvement in their ability to sustain attention and follow through on instructions following only limited practice of the procedure. Improvements were also noted for adults diagnosed with panic disorders that severely restricted their daily activities. The intensity of the panic attacks decreased immediately, and with continued practice of the procedure, the attacks eventually ceased.

The 4-D Formula

Even when energized and expanded, the aura is not always balanced and attuned. The 4-D Formula, another procedure utilizing the pyramid, is a comprehensive strategy designed to balance and attune not only the aura but the total person. This procedure emphasizes the totality of our being. The human aura is seen as a visible component within a multifaceted interactive systems. Consequently, balancing and attuning efforts that focus only on the aura are considered limited at best. This is not to minimize the importance of the visible aura, but rather to recognize the significant influence of other relevant facets, including mental, physical, and spiritual.

For this procedure, each of the pyramid's four sides symbolizes a critical dimension of the individual. With the pyramid positioned so that one side faces the subject, the left side represents the mind, the distant side represents the body, and the right side represents the spirit. The side of the pyramid facing the subject represents the subject's interactions with the other three sides. Here is the procedure:

Step 1. The Setting. Position the pyramid, with one side facing you, at a level to facilitate easy viewing.

Step 2. The Pyramid. Look at the pyramid, and think of it as an external model of your total being, with each side of the pyramid representing a critical dimension of yourself.

Step 3. The Mind. With your eyes closed, envision the left side of the pyramid and assign it the color yellow to signify the powers of your mind. Mentally divide that side of the pyramid into four levels, with each level representing one of four major mental elements: intelligence, memory, perception, and emotion. Assign a different tint of yellow, such as deep yellow for intelligence, medium yellow for memory, light yellow for perception, and very pale yellow for emotion. Finally, envision the four levels and their respective tints of yellow slowly merging to form a bright, swirling mixture of multi-tinted yellow energy. Sense the wondrous serenity and mental balance accompanying the merging of the powers of your mind.

Step 4. The Body. Think of the distant side of the pyramid as representing your physical body with its myriad of organs and systems. Mentally erect on that surface of the pyramid a variety of geometric designs-circles, squares, triangles, rectangles, and so forth. Assign the color of bright green to that side of the pyramid, with each geometric design of a different tint against a pale green background. Envision the isolated designs slowly gathering, while retaining their shapes, to engage a bright, kaleidoscopic pattern of interrelated green energy. Note the sense of physical balance and relaxation that accompanies the experience.

Step 5. The Spirit. Think of the right side of the pyramid as representing your spiritual being. Envision on that surface of the pyramid multiple shafts, each of a different tint of blue, crisscrossing in all directions like search lights against a pale blue background. Think of the multiple shafts as representing your spiritual interests and aspirations. A given shaft can symbolize your search for spiritual knowledge, and another, your altruistic strivings. Still others can represent your various spiritual growth needs. Envision the shafts interweaving and slowly coming together in a lattice pattern to form a multi-tinted blue spiral of bright, flowing energy. As each spiritual component contributes to the upward spiral of spiritual power, notice the wondrous infusion of energy throughout your total being.

Step 6. The Interaction. Focus your full attention on the side of the pyramid facing you. Envision pure cosmic energy being drawn from the center of the pyramid and displayed on the pyramid's front surface in a dynamic swirl of light. Then picture the cosmic swirl of pure energy as it draws multiple shades of yellow, green, and blue from the pyramid's other sides—filtering and illuminating them with pure cosmic energy to form a lustrous, colorful blend on the front surface of the pyramid. Finally, picture the cosmic swirl redistributing bright, cosmically charged energy throughout the pyramid. As you experience the new radiance of mental, physical, and spiritual energy represented by the pyramid, sense the powerful renewal within your own mind, body, and spirit. Your total energy system is now balanced and attuned—mentally, physically, and spiritually.

Step 7. Conclusion. To conclude the procedure, turn the palms of your hand toward the pyramid and sense its pulsating energies. With your eyes closed, envision the luminous energy of the pyramid entering your palms and spreading throughout your total being. Allow this energizing procedure to continue for several moments, then turn your hands upward and cross your lower arms to form an X. With your arms remaining crossed, bring them to your chest and rest your palms against your upper body. Notice the vibrant energy radiating from your palms, infusing and balancing your total being. Affirm, I am now balanced and attuned mentally, physically, and spiritually. I am at complete oneness with the cosmos.

Following this procedure, colors in the aura invariably become more radiant, and areas of discoloration tend to vanish. With repeated use of the procedure, voids in the aura become less pronounced, and eventually, they disappear altogether.

The Quartz Crystal

Like the pyramid, the quartz crystal is an all-purpose empowerment tool. It can be used as an induction tool for hypnosis and as a tangible cue to activate post-hypnotic suggestions. It can be incorporated as a tangible component into many structured empowerment strategies. There is strong evidence to indicate that it can be programmed to stimulate psychic development and promote success in achieving personal goals such as controlling weight, overcoming fears, and breaking unwanted habits. Our studies found that the crystal, when present in academic situations, can motivate students and improve test performance. When incorporated into various sports training programs, the quartz crystal can improve both individual and team performance. The quartz crystal is particularly effective in fine tuning the motor coordination skills required for many complex sports activities. Simply wearing the quartz crystal as a pendant is often sufficient to stimulate a peak performance.

Occasionally, the crystal will come into our lives spontaneously, as if to fulfill a special empowerment mission. A few years ago, a quartz crystal of unusual clarity and unique design inexplicably appeared on my office desk at Athens State University where I taught psychology and administered a parapsychology research program. The appearance of the crystal coincided with the near-depletion of crucial research funds. The survival of the parapsychology program was threatened, and several on-going research projects, including a critical study on altered states, were in jeopardy, with no new sources of funding in sight. Almost immediately following the appearance of the crystal, a major study on past-life regression was funded by the Parapsychology Foundation of New York. Soon afterward, additional parapsychology courses were introduced into the curriculum, and a million dollar parapsychology endowment drive was initiated. The crystal remained at its designated place until the college's parapsychology instructional and research programs were firmly established, whereupon it disappeared as mysteriously as it had appeared. Such a spontaneous phenomenon suggests the crystal is more than simply an object of beauty, it is possibly an instrument of power.

The empowerment effects of the crystal, like many other psychic tools, could be due either to the inherent power of the object itself or to the psychological associations we form with it. Our studies revealed that both factors working together are required to maximize the crystal's power. There is evidence to suggest that the crystal, like the pyramid, is empowering by its physical presence alone. But when we actively interact with the crystal, we expand its influence while stimulating the dormant powers within ourselves. Perhaps not surprising, then, the two essential components of all crystal empowerment strategies are: (1) recognizing the crystal's intrinsic empowerment potential, and (2) deliberately interacting with the crystal as an empowerment tool.

In our early laboratory studies of the crystal, we found that physical contact with the crystal alone, such as holding it in the hand, generated a calming effect among various physiological functions, including blood pressure and sweat gland activity. With appropriate orientation and the introduction of structured procedures, the calming effects of the crystal on the body markedly increased. Based on these findings, we developed several stress management strategies utilizing the crystal, including procedures for conquering stage fright, preventing panic attacks, improving concentration, and building self-confidence. Our later laboratory efforts focused on strategies that programmed the crystal to facilitate personal growth and achievement. Among the results of these studies are numerous laboratory-tested procedures for promoting career success, physical fitness, and self-improvement.

Our most recent research involving the crystal focused on its relevance to the human aura. Our studies consistently demonstrated the aura's high level of sensitivity to the crystal. Further study also revealed the crystal's high level of sensitivity, not only to the aura but to certain other critical factors, each of which we eventually incorporated into procedures designed to utilize this tool.

The effectiveness of the crystal as an aura empowerment tool depends on first, selecting an appropriate crystal, and second, effectively applying the crystal to achieve our empowerment goals. Three essential strategies—Crystal Scan, Crystal Programming, and Color Transfer—have been designed to maximize the effectiveness of the crystal as an aura empowerment tool. Crystal Scan is used as a selection technique, Crystal Programming is used as a goal-related strategy, and Color Transfer is used to add color to the aura following crystal programming.

Crystal Scan

Each crystal, like each human being, is a unique creation with its own individual characteristics. Crystals differ in their structural patterns as well as the quality and intensity of their vibrations. They also vary in the nature of their empowerment interactions with the human energy system. The ideal personal crystal is one that engages a strong empowerment response. But because our needs differ, there exist no perfect crystal for all our empowerment goals. A given crystal may be ideal for our health and fitness needs, whereas another crystal of markedly different features may be more effective for our career goals.

As a general rule, crystals that come to us as gifts are particularly empowering and are usually multi-purposeful. But for most of us, deciding to use the crystal for personal empowerment requires purposefully selecting an appropriate crystal from an assortment. Selecting a crystal from an assortment for personal use is usually a mutual process. The one that commands our attention or seems "to call out" to us is usually the ideal crystal for use at the time. The clear crystal seems to be suitable for most self-empowerment applications.

Crystal Scan is a crystal selection procedure that takes into consideration not only the general quality of our interaction with the crystal, but also the nature of our empowerment goals. Here is the strategy for selecting an appropriate crystal from an assortment.

Step 1. Goal Articulation. Definitively state your goal, and relate it to the crystal as an empowerment tool. Example: *My goal is to attune my aura system through interacting with the crystal as an empowerment tool.*

Step 2. Visual Scan. With your goal in mind, visually scan the assortment of crystals from left to right, a direction that seems to more readily discern the empowerment characteristics of crystals. Next, scan the assortment from right to left. Pay particular attention to crystals that assume a familiarity or command your attention.

Step 3. Sensate Scan. Place your hand a few inches over the assortment, and with the palm side down, slowly scan the assortment from left to right, then from right to left. As you reflect on your empowerment goal, sense the different energy frequencies emanating from the crystals and your interactions with them. Continue the sensate scan until a particular crystal emerges from the collection as ideally appropriate for your goal.

Step 4. Crystal Clasp. Upon sensing a certain crystal's receptiveness, clasp it in your hand and note its positive energies as confirmation of its appropriateness to your stated goal.

Crystal Programming

The crystal is more than a tool; it is a complex mechanism with interactive capacities and programming possibilities. When it comes to us spontaneously, it has probably been pre-programmed either generally or specifically for a particular purpose. Simply touching the crystal is usually sufficient to sense the harmony of its vibrations resulting from positive pre-programming.

After it is selected from an assortment, the crystal usually requires program unloading to clear out any residue of previous programming or surface accumulations of energy. This de-programming and clearing process is sometimes called "cleansing," a misnomer since the crystal is not "dirty," but rather a possible repository of extraneous frequencies or irrelevant energies. Program unloading is important because it ensures the crystal's optimal receptiveness to our empowerment programming efforts.

Several procedures have been proposed for deprogramming or clearing the crystal, some of which are rather intriguing. Examples are burying the crystal in moist sand, soaking it in either salt water or rain water, leaving it exposed to the elements for several days, exposing it overnight to the light of a full moon, and placing it in a vacuum. While these imaginative rituals may be quite effective, the key to crystal deprogramming is not in the ritual but in our interaction with the crystal during the deprogramming process. Not surprisingly, then, the most effective deprogramming will include a degree of physical and mental interaction with the crystal during the deprogramming effort. Simply running cool water over the crystal while holding and stroking it gently as your affirm your connection to it is an excellent deprogramming or clearing strategy.

Crystal programming actually begins when we select a receptive crystal and it continues as we deprogram it. Full programming of the crystal for a specific goal, however, requires a step-by-step, two-way interaction and the careful input of appropriate components. As a general rule, the clear crystal is more receptive to programming than crystals of color. We recommend the following programming procedure which is applied after the crystal has been appropriately deprogrammed.

Step 1. Programming Preliminaries. While holding the deprogrammed crystal loosely in your hand, think of it as your empowerment partner rather than simply an inert, intangible object. Observe its physical characteristics, especially its unique internal features. Close your eyes briefly and generate a detailed mental image of the crystal.

Step 2. Programming Interaction. Stroke the crystal gently and sense its energies. Note the positive interaction of your own energies with the crystal. Envision the energies emanating from the innermost part of the crystal as they unite with the energies emanating from the innermost part of your own being.

Step 3. Programming Dialogue. Articulate your empowerment objective by directly addressing the crystal and affirming: *Together, we will achieve (state your goal).* As you continue to hold the crystal, sense its receptivity to your stated goal.

Step 4. Final Affirmation. By programming the crystal, we re-affirm our empowerment goals and further commit ourselves to achieve them. Conclude the programming procedure with the simple affirmation: *I am empowered.*

As already noted, crystal programming is an interactive procedure. In programming the crystal as an empowerment partner, you are also programming yourself for success. The power of the crystal is always a function of our interactions with it. The programmed crystal, whether worn on the body or simply displayed for viewing, is an interactive partner in a mutual endeavor.

Whatever the nature of our goals, certain effects of crystal programming are usually visible immediately in the aura system. Three crucial changes suggesting a significant energizing effect almost always occur: (1) the aura's inner regions become increasingly bright, (2) the aura's outer region expands, and (3) subtle changes in coloration emerge.

The immediate effects of crystal programming on the aura set the stage for continued interactions with the crystal and additional changes in the aura related to the stated empowerment goals. Aside from the immediate effects, certain goal-related changes will spontaneously unfold as the result of initial programming and thus, will require no additional effort. But fully maximizing the power of crystal programming usually requires supplemental strategies and additional goal-related intervention.

As we already know, color in the aura is a manifestation of energy, with each color variation designating a particular energy function. As expected, the spontaneous color changes resulting from crystal programming typically relate to the empowerment goals. They are seen as either restorative or additive in nature rather than drastic modifications to the aura system. They meet deficiencies, correct malfunctions, and restore the aura's energy resources. We found that when the coloration changes were finally complete, the empowerment goals had almost always been realized.

In our laboratory, the spontaneous changes in aura coloration resulting from Crystal Programming were found to be consistent with our previous observations that related color in the aura to certain personal characteristics. Not surprisingly, programming related to health goals typically added bright green. Social and career-related programming, on the other hand, usually introduced a bright shade of yellow into the aura. Programming focusing on rejuvenation goals almost always generated a new layer of pink in the inner region of the aura; whereas programming designed to balance and attune the aura usually extracted discoloration and added a layer of iridescent blue to the middle region of the aura.

Programming designed to protect the aura system often produces a thin but powerful shield of gleaming white energy that envelops the total aura. The shield protects the energy system from any invasion of negative forces that could damage the aura or deplete its energy supply. Although the shield is impervious to external threat, it does not inhibit our capacity to interact with other energy sources, including other aura systems.

The long-term effects of Crystal Programming on the aura depend on the programming goals. For short-term goals, programming can be highly successful but transient. For instance, an important career-related task or a crisis situation may require a temporary abundance of specialized energy. When the task is complete or the crisis is resolved, the aura's energy level returns to normal. On the other hand, long-term goals involving personal growth and commitment may require permanent changes in the aura's structure and functions.

Color Transfer

Color Transfer is a supplemental strategy designed to maximize the effects of Crystal Programming by using the same programmed crystal to enrich the aura with additional energy related to the empowerment goal. The procedure was developed in our laboratories following our observations of spontaneous changes in the aura's color make-up resulting from Crystal Programming. Crystal Transfer holds that various energy forms, each with a different color, are transferable from the programmed crystal to the aura. The strategy is implemented only after the spontaneous color changes resulting from Crystal Programming are clearly visible in the aura. The color added through the procedure is always consistent with the color changes already underway in the visible aura. The procedure requires viewing the aura and then uses imagery to visualize the color emanating from the crystal as a specialized manifestation of energy, poised for transfer to the aura system.

Step 1. **Aura Perception.** View your personal aura using the Psychic Self-perception Procedure as previously presented in Chapter 3. Focus your attention on the unfinished work in your aura. Examples are a void not yet filled or a new band of color not yet complete.

Step 2. **Goal Affirmation.** With the programmed crystal resting in your hand, review your empowerment goal and reaffirm your commitment to achieve it.

Step 3. **Energy Perception.** Sense the energy emanating from the crystal. Visualize the color manifestation of the energy and sense your own energy system interacting with it.

Step 4. **Energy Transfer.** As you envision your aura, think of the regions undergoing change as construction sites. Visualize colorful energy from the crystal being channeled to your aura. Establish a steady flow of energy between the crystal and the work sites in your aura.

Step 5. Goal Re-affirmation. Relate the flow of energy between the crystal and your aura to your stated goal. Again, reaffirm your goal and your power to achieve it.

Step 6. Power Reinforcement. Reinforce the energy interaction by periodically stroking the crystal as you envision the channel connecting you to it. Sense the continuous flow of energy between the crystal and your energy system.

It is of paramount importance to again emphasize that Color Transfer is used only with an appropriately programmed crystal.

Gems

As objects of beauty and value, gems have assumed empowering significance among many cultures. They are often associated with the finest expression of human emotions, including love, commitment, honor, and celebration. Ironically, gems can also evoke the darkest side of human conduct—envy, greed, and exploitation. Misfortune and tragic death are often seen in the history of rare and famous gems. Regardless of a gem's monetary value or provenance, it remains simply a tangible object. From the psychic empowerment perspective, gems are empowering only when they facilitate the growth process.

Unlike the quartz crystal, the energy design of precious and semi-precious gems is relatively if not fully fixed and, consequently, not typically receptive to programming. Nevertheless, many gems seem to possess significant empowerment potential. Certain gems, for instance, appear innately empowering in their capacity to spontaneously interact with the human aura. But other gems require structured procedures to access and activate their empowerment capacities. Still other gems are empowering due primarily to their psychological significance, including the effects of the associations we form with them. Whatever the nature of the gem, our expectations of it as an empowerment tool is a decisive force affecting its empowerment potential. That influence can generate significant empowerment results independent of the gem's natural characteristics. As a general rule, the gem's empowerment effects are greatest when the gem is physically present or worn.

Emerald

As a power tool, the emerald is recognized primarily for its rejuvenating properties. It may seem improbable that a simple gem could influence the complex mental and physical dynamics of aging. Nonetheless, the emerald, by its physical presence alone, seems to do just that. In our surveys of centenarians, the emerald was found to be their number one gem of preference. Although they seldom attributed their longevity solely to the gem, centenarians often reported a long, positive association with it, typically as an adornment. Among our many survey respondents was the owner of a retail chain who, at age 103, reported feeling "not fully dressed" unless wearing her trademark emerald brooch. Along a similar line, a business owner attributed both his excellent health and career success to an emerald tie-pin given him at an early age by his father. At age 101, he continues to wear the emerald daily, claiming it always brings him good fortune.

Based on a comprehensive analysis of many reports concerning the special rejuvenating properties of the emerald, we developed the Emerald Rejuvenation Procedure, an age management approach designed to link the emerald's rejuvenation properties to the power within ourselves to influence the normal aging process. Aura viewings before and after the procedure reveal significant changes in both brightness and coloration. Typically, the aura's inner region becomes illuminated with shimmering emerald-green energy.

The procedure recognizes three crucial possibilities for managing aging: first, the emerald is independently capable, as a tangible object, of directly influence aging; second, we possess within ourselves the power to slow, arrest, and even reverse aging; and third, by interacting with the emerald, we can activate both of these power sources, thereby unleashing abundant rejuvenating energy with the potential to arrest and even reverse aging.

Step 1. Rejuvenation Touch. Touch the emerald and sense its energies. Let your energy frequencies interact with those of the emerald. Note the nature of the emerald's frequencies and your mental and physical interactions with them.

Step 2. Energy Dispersion. With your eyes closed, hold the emerald and sense its emission of energy fully saturating your physical body. Slowly absorb the emerald's flow of energy into the deeper regions of your body.

Step 3. Rejuvenation Imagery. As you continue to hold the emerald, envision yourself at your youthful prime, perhaps standing disrobed before a full-length mirror. Sense the emerald's energy enveloping your body with a youthful glow, gently erasing all physical signs of aging.

Step 4. Concluding Affirmation. Conclude the procedure by affirming: *I am infused with healthful, rejuvenating energy. By simply touching the emerald, I can at any moment activate its rejuvenating power.*

In addition to rejuvenation, this strategy is also valued for its health enhancing effects. We can evaluate the immediate results of the procedure by viewing the aura using any of the previously discussed hand-viewing techniques before and after the exercise. Frequent physical contact with the emerald ensures an uninterrupted flow of rejuvenating energy.

Amethyst

The amethyst gem is noted for its mental and physical health properties. It appears to balance the aura system and promote a healthy mind/body interaction. It tends to add shades of pink or rose to the aura, particularly around the head, shoulders, and chest. Its energies can be targeted to specific areas of the aura, depending on our physical or mental health needs. Discoloration in the aura associated with physical and mental distress can be discharged through clearing and stabilizing strategies that utilize the amethyst.

In addition to its healthful energies, the amethyst is sometimes associated with psychic growth and wisdom. As a psychic empowerment tool, it has been highly effective when incorporated into programs designed to develop various psychic faculties. In our laboratory, it demonstrated particular effectiveness in stimulating PK. Many advanced health and fitness programs recognize the PK power of the mind to influence biological functions. The unusual effectiveness of the amethyst as a health and wellness tool may be largely due to its usefulness in activating the mind's PK capacity to promote healthy biological functioning.

The Amethyst Power Strategy, which was developed in our laboratories and used in our health and fitness programs, is based on a three-fold premise: First, awaiting our self-discovery is a vast inner region of health and fitness potential; second, the mind holds supreme power over the body with capacity to unleash abundant health and fitness energy; and finally, the amethyst as an empowerment tool can effectively interact with our total energy system to activate our dormant inner resources. The effects of the gem on the aura are usually long-term because of its capacity to strengthen the aura's basic structure.

Step 1. Interacting Through Touch. While holding the amethyst in either hand, focus your full attention on its various characteristics, including color, weight, and temperature. Sense the vibrations of its energies, and its interactions with your aura system. Transfer the amethyst to your other hand, and note again your interactions with it.

Step 2. Praying Hands Energy Exchange. Bring your hands together in the praying hands position with the amethyst resting between your palms. Sense the exchange of energies occurring between your hands and the amethyst. Notice your sense of renewal as abundant energy spreads throughout your physical body.

Step 3. Solar Plexus Empowerment. Focus your attention on the energy core in your solar plexus, now pulsating with power and diffusing bright new energy and vitality into your surrounding aura.

Step 4. Energy Balancing. Envision the amethyst between your hands as it actively balances you mentally, physically, and spiritually. Sense the expiation of all negative influences and the clearing of any discoloration in your aura system. Focus on specific dysfunctional areas and bathe them with healing energy.

Step 5. Concluding Affirmation. Conclude the procedure by affirming: *All the systems of my being are balanced and attuned. I am infused with healthful energy. Mentally, physically, and spiritually, I am fully empowered.*

As with the emerald, the effects of the amethyst on the aura can be assessed by hand-viewing strategies applied before and after the procedure. Frequent contact with the amethyst tends to amplify its energies and reinforce its specialized effects.

Topaz

The dynamics associated with the topaz are similar to those of the amethyst with one exception—the topaz is highly specialized in its capacity to target empowering energy to the body's immune system. It introduces a shimmering glow into the aura, typically in the form of a bright sheath enveloping the body at the innermost region of the visible aura. Regular physical contact with the topaz, either as a pendant or ring, sustains the sheath and its power to safeguard the body's immune system.

The power of the topaz can be maximized through a simple strategy that visualizes its functions and affirms its capacity to empower the immune system. Here is the procedure:

Step 1. Topaz Partnership. Establish a partnership with the topaz by wearing it as a pendant or ring for a few days. Sense your evolving attachment to the topaz, and give it your consent to protect your body by building your resistance to illness.

Step 2. Topaz Touch. Hold the topaz between your hands and sense its vibrations. Envision bright energy radiating from the gem to form a bright shield around your physical body. Think of the gem as a health and fitness partner with abundant protective resources. Affirm: *I am empowered by the healthful energies emanating from this gem.*

Step 3. Aura Viewing. Using any of the hand-viewing strategies previously discussed, view your aura and note the glistening shield of energy around your hand.

Step 4. Affirmation of Partnership. Reaffirm your partnership with the topaz as a tool for empowering your immune system.

Although the topaz is an important health enhancing tool, it is not a replacement for a healthful life style. A balanced diet, exercise, recreation, safe sex, and a positive outlook remain among the essential components of any effective health and fitness plan.

Sapphire

The sapphire exists in all colors of the rainbow, but the best known variety of this gem has blue tints. The star sapphire is characterized by a crystal structure that reflects light in star-like rays. Sapphires with this characteristic, called *asterism,* are noted for their capacity to introduce an ethereal purity into the aura.

As a psychic empowerment tool, the sapphire is typically associated with love, affection, and compassion. In our survey of college students, men and women who identified the sapphire as their favorite gem, or the gem they would most likely wear, were typically pursuing careers in the so-called helping professions, including teaching, psychology, social work, and counseling. Almost never did natural science, engineering, and business majors specify the sapphire as their favorite gem.

The sapphire is often seen as an important link to the universe. In its capacity for cosmic resonance, the sapphire is believed to amplify the aura, and promote a state of cosmic attunement. Areas of discord in the aura are brought into harmony with the inner-self and the cosmos. Among the psychological effects associated with this gem are security feelings, self-confidence, and a heightened state of mental alertness.

When present, the sapphire usually introduces a degree brightness into the aura, an effect that seems to occur independent of any deliberate effort on our part. But when incorporated into an appropriate procedure, the sapphire produces a very brilliant, luminous glow throughout the aura with sparkling blue rays that seem to radiate outward from the aura's central energy core.

The Sapphire Star Procedure was developed to boost the spontaneous functions of the sapphire as an empowerment tool. The procedure recognizes the sapphire's long history as a love charm, but focuses primarily on the gem's relevance to psychological empowerment and cosmic attunement.

Step 1. Touch. With the sapphire resting in your hand, notice the various features of the gem, particularly its coloration. Gently stroke the gem and sense its energies.

Step 2. Physical Interaction. As you continue to hold the gem, close your eyes and envision the bright, star-like energy radiating from it. Sense your interaction with the gem and its energies. Note the tranquil effects of the gem on your physical body.

Step 3. Auric Interaction. Sense the inner core of your aura interacting with the sapphire to produce crystal blue energy that illuminates your total aura. Envision brilliant rays of blue energy extending to the outermost reaches of your aura.

Step 4. Cosmic Interaction. Envision a higher cosmic dimension of power with its brilliant core generating radiant energy as powerful shafts that interact with your own energy system. Note the wondrous sense of new power and balance within your total being.

Step 5. Empowerment Affirmation. Again stroke the sapphire and affirm: *I am infused with new power and attuned to the universe.* You may wish to wear the sapphire as a constant reminder and manifestation of your contact with the cosmic source of pure energy.

Your can observe the physical effects of this procedure on your aura by using the Aura Hand-viewing Strategy previously discussed. Notice particularly the rays of bright blue energy reaching into the outer regions of the aura. Since the aura around your hand is fairly representative of your full aura, the Aura Hand-viewing Strategy can immediately evaluate the effects of the procedure on your total aura system.

These are only a few examples of gems as potential empowerment tools. You may be surprised to note that we did not included the diamond among our empowering gems. Unlike other gems, the diamond, which is the hardest substance in nature, appears to possess few if any empowering properties. Although it is promoted in our culture as a symbol of undying love and commitment, our research suggested, to our surprise, that this costly gem is, in fact, often disempowering. Our laboratory studies using biofeedback technology yielded measures suggesting increased stress and physical enfeebling effects when the diamond was introduced into the experimental situation. Strength of grip as measured by a hand dynamometer (Lafayette Instrument Co.) dropped an average of five kilograms for men and seven kilograms for women when a diamond was held for five minutes in the hand prior to measuring the hand's strength of grip. After prolonged contact with the diamond, the strength of grip dropped even further. On another laboratory task using a rotometer to measure steadiness of hand, holding a stylus on a moving target became increasingly difficult with the introduction of the diamond.

Many professional athletes have inadvertently discovered the diamond's tendency to deplete their energy supply and interfere with their performance, particularly in activities requiring endurance and technical excellence. In sports activities ranging from gymnastics to auto racing, the diamond can be decisive in negatively tilting the performance scales. Balance, concentration, and motor coordination are especially vulnerable to the diamond's influence. The cumulative effects of the diamond in athletics can literally increase the probability of physical injury and mistakes in judgment.

The influence of the diamond is readily visible in the human aura. Typically, the surrounding energy field becomes constricted, and the brightness in aura coloration increasingly diminishes. The diamond accentuates dysfunctional areas in the aura and makes self-intervention efforts more difficult.

Fabrics

We are a fashion conscious culture. Magazines devoted primarily to fashion trends are among the most popular. We learn at an early age to value designer apparel and contemporary styles. When fashions change, we change with them. Trendiness in attire remains at or near the top of our scale of values.

Aside from its cultural significance, our personal attire can have important psychological impact. A new garment can temporarily give us an emotional lift and increase our sense of personal worth. The important events in our lives are often punctuated and later remembered by the clothing we wore for the occasion. In our past-life regression studies, among the first things to command our subjects' attention as they experienced their past lives were the color, style, and fabric of their clothing. Even non-distinctive styles and drab colors do not escaped the discriminating eye during regression. The images of apparel seem to linger as significant messengers out of the past.

While the cultural and psychological significance of clothing is commonly recognized, the impact of apparel on the human aura system has received only scant attention. In our studies, we found that the aura is particularly sensitive to fabrics and their colors. As previously noted, many aura specialists contend that the ideal, though not always practical, condition for accurate aura viewing requires a disrobed subject because of the influence of one's clothing on the visible aura. We also noted, however, that the skilled aura viewer is usually able to recognize the influence of clothing on the aura and thus screen it out during viewing.

Our studies found that the effects of apparel on the aura can be either positive or negative, depending on the nature of the fabric and our interaction with it. Although fiber sensitivity levels vary from person to person (and from aura to aura), natural fibers and their blends, including cotton, silk, wool, and linen, tend to energize and add brightness to the aura, whereas synthetics and synthetic blends tend to either constrict or agitate the aura.

In addition to fabric sensitivity, certain auras are highly color sensitive. The predominantly orange aura is among the most highly color sensitive, particularly to the warm colors and certain shades of green. The rainbow and predominantly light blue auras, on the other hand, are usually non-color sensitive. Top fashion models almost always have either rainbow or predominantly light blue auras which are complemented by apparel of any color or color combination. As a general rule, fabric colors that enhance our physical appearance are likewise enhancing to the aura. Blue, white, and off-white fabrics are usually compatible to auras of any color.

The effects of fabrics, including both fiber and color, obviously extend to sleeping apparel and bed coverings. In our sleep studies, sleeping apparel and bed coverings of cotton or silk, in either white, off-white, or pale blue, were found to be compatible to auras of any color or energy frequency. Dark fabrics, especially synthetics and synthetic blends, were found to be typically less conducive to sleep than pastel shades. Black, dark brown, and red fabrics, whether natural or synthetic, were found to be almost always disruptive to sound sleep.

Since the interaction between the aura and apparel is usually immediate, any of the aura hand-viewing techniques can be used to assess the effects of the interaction on the aura system. In selecting a garment for wear, simply draping it over the bare arm as the aura around the hand is viewed can provide a useful assessment of our interaction with the garment. This simple test is particularly important when purchasing garments. The ideal garment will complement the aura rather than detract from it. Garments that clash with the aura should be rejected, since their disruptive effects are cumulative and can only increase as we wear the garment. Most of us have inadvertently selected an inharmonious garment and, having worn it only briefly, experienced its negative influence on our energy system (and we may have hung it in a closet never to wear it again). Reactions such as fatigue, tension, and even illness can result from prolonged exposure to garments that are incompatible with the aura.

Our findings concerning the effects of fibers and colors on the human energy system have important implications for the home and work environment. By taking into consideration the nature of the human aura, commercial and residential buildings can be designed to enrich our interactions and empower our lives. As a general rule, a spacious, open, uncluttered living and work space which complements and integrates the surrounding natural environment is empowering to the human aura and conducive to productive interactions. The optimal building structure and decor consists of natural materials, with wood, stone, marble, metal, glass, and natural fibers preferred over plastics, synthetics, and other human-made materials. Synthetic carpeting is particularly enfeebling to auras which are highly sensitive to fabrics.

Dowsing

Without a consideration of dowsing, our study of aura empowerment tools would be incomplete. Dowsing as it relates to the human aura is primarily an assessment procedure consisting of three major applications: (1) The procedure can identify problem areas by scanning the immediate aura; (2) it can chart the outer, invisible borders of the aura system; and (3) it can assess the developmental nature of the aura's frequency patterns. For these applications, dowsing requires L-shaped metal rods which are held parallel, one in each hand, with the longer segment (approximately twelve inches) pointed forward and carefully balanced along the index finger to permit easy, unobstructed movement. When sleeves are used for the shorter hand-held segments, they should be metal rather than plastic which can inhibit the recording capacity of the rods.

As an assessment or recording procedure, dowsing is based on the premise that different energy systems exist with regions and boundaries that are sensitive to our probes. Among the most intimate of these energy systems is the human aura. Using metal rods as extensions of physiology, experienced dowsers can identify, chart, and assess the energies surrounding the subject's physical body.

The Aura Dowsing Procedure

Dowsing as applied to the aura is typically used in conjunction with aura viewing strategies. Since the visible aura is considered only a limited representation of the total aura system, dowsing can be used to identify certain aspects of its unseen features, including its distant boundaries. Although the energies of the human aura can conceivably stretch to infinity, the immediate aura system consists of identifiable concentric regions with distinct perimeters, seven of which are usually detectable through dowsing.

In addition to detecting the boundaries of the aura's concentric regions, dowsing can accurately assess the frequency patterns of each region. This procedure usually requires practice in sensing and comparing the aura frequency patterns of many individuals.

The *Aura Dowsing Procedure* is an assessment and diagnostic strategy that uses dowsing to analyze the aura's immediate and extended design, including both structural and functional characteristics.

Step 1. Aura Viewing. With your subject standing, view the aura using any of the aura viewing procedures previously discussed.

Step 2. Localized Aura Scan. This step consists of three phases:

(I) **Frontal Scan.** While facing your subject, use metal L-shaped dowsing rods, one held in each hand, to scan the aura immediately surrounding your subject's physical body. Begin at the head region with a rod held to each side of the subject at a few inches from the body. Slowly progress downward as you sense any problem areas or abrupt changes in energy frequencies being recorded by the rods. Conduct a second face-to-face scan, again noting the aura's unique energy characteristics. Record your findings on the Aura Map and Analysis Form (see Figure 6, page 179).

(II) **Side Scan.** Change your position to facing either side of your subject, and again scan the aura from the head downward, with one rod held a few inches to the front of your subject and the other rod held a few inches to the back. As in the face-to-face scan, note any changes in energy frequencies and patterns. Repeat the scan as you again note its unique characteristics. Record your findings on the Aura Map and Analysis Form.

(III) **Scan Comparison.** Compare the results of the frontal and side scans, giving particular attention to overall energy patterns and specific frequency characteristics.

Step 3. Regional Border Scan. This step consists of two phases:

(I) Sequential Scans. Beginning at a distance of approximately twenty-five feet from your subject, and with the rods pointed directly toward your subject, slowly move forward until the rods spread apart, a signal that you have approached the perimeter of an outer energy region. On the floor, mark the border with either tape or chalk. Step just inside the marked perimeter and with the rods pointed toward your subject, slowly move forward until the rods separate again, a signal that you have reached the second perimeter in the subjects energy system. As before, mark the border with tape or chalk. Repeat the regional border scans until you reach the innermost perimeter, which is usually around 12 to 18 inches from your subject.

(II) Repeat Scan(s). Repeat the full scan procedure in order to confirm the perimeters identified by your first scan. You will probably note small discrepancies in the scans, a phenomenon due primarily to the fluid nature of the aura system. In cases of serious discrepancies, conduct additional scans until you reach a reasonable consensus.

Step 4. Analysis. Measure the distance of each perimeter from your subject, then chart the scan results on the Aura Map and Analysis Form. Compare the results of the regional and localized scans and relate them to your earlier viewing of the aura. The highly developed aura system will usually have a freely detectable region of energy at a distance of around twenty feet, with the remaining perimeters readily evident. The less highly developed aura system will have a more constricted energy field with less clearly defined perimeters. On average, the concentric regions of the aura system will progressively weaken as they extended away from the subject.

Step 5. Empowerment Interaction. This step is designed to promote an empowering interaction with your subject by providing a positive interpretation of the scan results with emphasis

AURA MAP AND ANALYSIS FORM

Name of Subject:
Date of Birth:
Date of Viewing: Place of Viewing: Viewer:

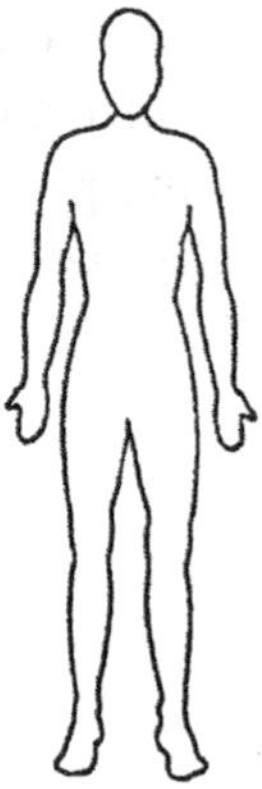

Coloration Patterns:

Structural Features and Designs:

Frequency Characteristics:

Comments and Conclusions:

FIGURE 6. AURA MAP AND ANALYSIS FORM.

on the growth potentials and empowerment possibilities uncovered by the procedure. Using non-evaluative strategies, suggest relevant empowerment options available to your subject, including appropriate self-intervention procedures.

Summary

Our study of psychic tangibles provides important evidence of the abounding power and remarkable resiliency of the human aura. We have found that the aura is receptive to empowerment tangibles that range from trees to gems. When incorporated into appropriate procedures, psychic tangibles become powerful tools that connect us, not only to the power within ourselves, but to the highest powers of the cosmos.

8

The Interactive Aura

You are, when all is done—just what you are.

—Goethe, "Faust's Study,"
from *Faust: Part I*
(1808)

A S HUMAN BEINGS, we are the totality of our mental, physical, and spiritual interactions, which can reach from our closest reality to the most distant reaches of the cosmos. In addition to the on-going interactions within ourselves, we interact with others through our thoughts, feelings, and actions. We interact with our physical surroundings through our sensory processes—sight, hearing, smell, taste, and touch. Through our extrasensory faculties, we interact with realities that lie beyond our sensory thresholds. Psychically and spiritually, we interact with intangible dimensions and non-temporal sources of limitless power. Angels, ministering spirits, discarnate entities, and higher astral planes are all within the scope of our interactive powers.

Because of its acute sensitivity and adaptive capacity, the human aura is a critical component of our interactive nature. The aura is, in fact, an interactive system. It spontaneously transforms our experiences, including our emotions, thoughts, and interactions, into visible energy manifestations. As we know already, positive experiences tend to expand and illuminate the aura. It logically follows that positive self-interactions are among the most effective ways of empowering and energizing the aura. All the tools and strategies of psychic empowerment are built around the centerpiece of positive human expression, including thought, imagery, affirmation, and action.

In contrast to the positive experiences that empower the aura, negative experiences tend to constrict and drain it of energy, effects that are readily visible in the aura. Negative self-expressions, such as hostility, resentment, ill-will, worry, agitation, and hopelessness, invariably weaken and discolor the aura. Furthermore, the same influences that disempower the aura likewise disempower the mind, body, and spirit. A major goal of psychic empowerment is to reverse the disempowerment effects of our negative self-expressions by uncovering our positive resources and using them to empower our lives.

Like the interactions within the self, external conditions can also interact with the aura to influence its functions. As we have seen, our interactions with the tangibles around us, particularly our natural surroundings, can empower not only to the aura, but the mind, body, and spirit as well. They can lift us to new levels of awareness and give new meaning to our lives. Similarly, our interactions with the spiritual realm can directly empower the aura while instilling within us a deeper understanding of our existence. We emerge from these interactions enlightened, inspired, energized, and attuned, effects which are immediately reflected in the aura.

Among the most critical conditions influencing the aura are our interactions with others. Positive social interactions, whether with individuals or within groups, typically energize, expand, and illuminate our surrounding energy field. In the group setting, positive interactions can literally generate an extended body of bright energy that can often be seen hovering above the group, a synergistic phenomenon that can be felt by anyone joining the group or entering the space occupied by the group, even after the group has dispersed. Negative social interactions, on the other hand, tend to constrict, deplete, and discolor the aura. None of us is invulnerable to adverse social influences. Examples are betrayal and deception that generate distrust and anguish, negative encounters that distract us and impair our ability to constructively focus our energies, and fractured relationships that exact a painful toll on our adjustment resources. But when facing adversity, it is important to keep in mind that even negative experiences can be turned into growth opportunities. They challenge us to face adversity and rise above it. A strong, empowered aura will invariably reflect the growth benefits of past adversity.

Social influences are often so subtle that they escape our conscious awareness. They can be evident, nevertheless, in not only the aura but our behavior as well. In our person-to-person interactions, for instance, we spontaneously adjust the spatial distance between ourselves and the other person, a subtle phenomenon which seems to parallel the interaction of the two energy systems. Simply put, we literally move toward people whose energies attract us and away from people whose energies repel us. We typically make no effort to adjust spatial distance when the energies are neutral.

Visual inspection of the aura during positive social interactions typically reveals highly energized, expansive systems suggesting mutual attraction. The auras in such relationships seem to reach out, connect, and in some instances, literally embrace. Conversely, mutually negative interactions typically result in constricted auras with a space barrier between them.

In couples counseling, the auras of an alienated couple can be seen literally repelling each other and resisting interaction. Almost without exception, changes in the two auras effectively monitor the couple's progress, or lack of it, in resolving problems in the relationship. Among couples as well as groups, mutually satisfying interactions usually generate radiant energy throughout the auras of all participants. Many of the aura empowerment strategies previously discussed, such as the Cosmic Centering Procedure and the Comprehensive Intervention Strategy, can be easily adapted to couples and groups. Simply participating in aura viewing exercises can energize the aura and generate productive social interactions. Also, various empowerment tangibles and their related strategies, such as the Empowerment Walk, Tree Power Interaction, and Pyramid of Power as previously discussed, are highly effective when practiced by couples and groups.

Mutually positive energy interactions exercise the empowered aura's capacity not only to generate energy, but to send and receive it as well. The already empowered aura is energized further by positive exchanges with other aura systems. The enfeebled or underdeveloped aura with deficient energy, on the other hand, is often unable to generate, let alone send energy. For individuals who have not mastered effective self-energizing strategies, a one-way energy infusion from others may seem to be the only source of renewed energy. These individuals may consequently seek out highly energized persons with abundant, overflowing energy, or persons who, by nature, are nurturing and giving. The result can be either alienation from persons who are not nurturing or a dependent relationship with persons who are nurturing. Occasionally, a co-dependent relationship will develop in which persons with the need to nurture depend on persons with the need to be nurtured, and vice versa. The long-term effects of these relationships are often arrested growth for both participants.

Psychic Vampirism

Occasionally, the underdeveloped aura system with deficient energy resources will acquire an adaptive pattern of habitually invading the aura systems of others and drawing energy from them. This phenomenon, which we previously referred to as psychic vampirism for lack of a better term, results in an immediate surge of new energy for the so-called psychic vampire and a marked depletion of energy for the host victim. Although the typical vampire interaction will last only minutes at most, the residual effects on the victim, which can include dizziness, loss of energy, muscle tension, difficulty concentrating, headaches, and nausea, can last for days. Repeated vampire attacks can lead to chronic fatigue, sleep disturbances, irritability, depressed mood, and even physical illness in the host victim.

Psychic vampirism is probably far more widespread that is generally realized. We have all experienced social interactions that seemed to drain us of our energies, and we may know individuals who habitually tire or wear down people around them. Even during brief, casual encounters, the experienced psychic vampire can lock into our energy system and rapidly exhaust our energy resources. Though we may not have attributed our energy loss in these situations to psychic vampirism, we probably became somewhat more guarded in similar future interactions.

As a group, psychic vampires are quite varied in their personal traits and behavioral patterns. Many of them fit the so-called "smooth operator" stereotype. They are sometimes without scruples, and can stoop to almost any means to meet their energy needs. They can appear passive and reserved, effectively disguising any inclination toward vampirism, but when the situation demands it, they can be overly assertive and even intimidating. They may actively prey on the vulnerabilities of others, poised to strike at the opportune moment, or they may manipulate their target victim through claims of special gifts or powers. In the work setting, they are usually difficult to work with. They are usually inconsistent in their job performance, often alternating between high efficiency and total ineffectiveness.

Despite their disguises, psychic vampires are typically insecure and vulnerable. Although they may display an air of self-importance, they operate from a position of weakness, not power. They usually have limited insight into themselves, and they are quick to pass judgments on people around them. They often complain about being treated unfairly, while at the same time, they are characteristically self-centered and inconsiderate of others. Their personal relationships are typically unstable. Many of them meet the criteria for a personality disorder, with such symptoms as emotional insecurity, difficulty controlling anger, poor self-image, and a weak sense of self. They often harbor smoldering hostility, which from time to time, will explode in an outburst of anger. They are found in all career settings, including colleges and universities where, as self-anointed "scholars," they have been known to overstate their academic qualifications. Pseudo-intellectuals and the so-called "expert debunkers" of psychic phenomena seem especially prone to psychic vampirism.

The vampire interaction can be either deliberate or spontaneous on the part of the vampire, and consensual or non-consensual on the part of the host victim. The typical vampire attack is probably spontaneous, thus requiring little or no conscious effort to initiate or maintain it. In many spontaneous interactions, neither the victim nor the vampire is aware that energy transfer is occurring. Although the victim is typically in the vampire's range of peripheral vision, the attack itself may involve little or no eye contact.

Many psychic vampires, upon becoming cognizant of their vampire tendencies, rationalize them as acceptable forms of needs fulfillment. They deliberately plan their vampire rendezvous as they would other social engagements. Their tactics are designed to transiently engage the unsuspecting partner in a spatially close interaction during which the unexpected attack occurs. Psychic vampires often use blatant flattery, excessive friendliness, undue generosity, and a measured degree of self-disclosure to captivate their victim and maintain the interaction for the duration of the attack.

Casual vampire attacks, in contrast to the planned attack, often involve little or no preliminary social interaction with the victim, who may be deliberately selected solely on the basis of availability. The causal attack is usually inconspicuous with the victim oblivious to the invasion. The results are, nonetheless, the same as for a planned attack—the vampire is satiated and the unwitting victim is depleted a measure of energy. These casual exchanges can occur almost anywhere—a classroom, office, restaurant, plane, gym, or any public gathering.

Psychic Vampirism in the Laboratory

Like other behavioral patterns, psychic vampirism exists on a continuum. While almost everyone can possess at least some of the characteristics associated with psychic vampirism, this does not mean that they are active psychic vampires. Only when the tendencies associated with vampirism become sufficient to interfere with one's own well-being or the well-being of others can the individual be considered an active psychic vampire.

In our laboratory, we developed two questionnaires for assessing psychic vampirism, not as a disorder but as a set of behavioral traits or tendencies. Interaction Questionnaire I evaluates psychic vampirism in one's relationship to people in general. Interaction

Questionnaire II evaluates psychic vampirism in one's relationship to a particular partner. Both questionnaires, which can be self-administered, make no direct reference to psychic vampirism.

Interaction Questionnaire I

Name:_____ Age:____ Gender:_____

Directions: This questionnaire is designed to assess certain aspects of your interactions with others. Read each statement carefully. If the statement is true as applied to you, circle T. If the statement is false as applied to you, circle F.

T F   1. I am attracted to people who are full of energy.

T F   2. I often call upon people to do things for me that I could do for myself.

T F   3. I usually get the things I want one way or another.

T F   4. When I am low, I become energized by simply being around people.

T F   5. I usually get restless when not traveling around or being involved with people.

T F   6. At times I find satisfaction in taking advantage of people who leave themselves open to it.

T F   7. I often make friends because they are useful to me in some way.

T F   8. I often do risky things just for the thrill of it.

T F   9. At times I experience a fascinating connection to a total stranger.

T F 10. I tend to thrive on the energies of people around me.

To score the questionnaire, simply count the number of T responses (F responses have no score value). A total score of 1 to 5 indicates no significant psychic vampirism; 6 to 8 indicates mild psychic vampirism; 8 to 9 indicates moderate psychic vampirism; and 10 indicates severe psychic vampirism. Items 6 and 10 on this questionnaire were found to be key predictors of psychic vampirism. Our analysis found that respondents who answered T to either of these items almost invariably scored in the severe range of psychic vampirism.

To assess psychic vampirism in a partner relationship, Interaction Questionnaire II as follows is administered to both partners. The scoring and interpreting procedures are the same as for Interaction Questionnaire I.

Interaction Questionnaire II

Name:_____ Age:____ Gender:_____

Directions: This questionnaire is designed to assess certain aspects of your interactions with others. Read each statement carefully. If the statement is true as applied to you, circle T. If the statement is false as applied to you, circle F.

T F 1. I can usually persuade my partner to see things my way.

T F 2. I become energized by being around my partner.

T F 3. I tend to be manipulative or controlling in my relationship with my partner.

T F 4. I find satisfaction in having a certain power over my partner.

T F 5. My partner often complains of low energy or fatigue.

T F 6. My partner seems to avoid me at times.

T F 7. I often call on my partner for help with things I could easily do for myself.

T F 8. I tend to become restless when separated for a few days from my partner.

T F 9. If separated from my partner for a prolonged period, I would probably seek out another partner with whom to interact.

T F 10. I probably receive more than I give in my relationship with my partner.

On this questionnaire, Items 3 and 10 were found to be key predictors of severe psychic vampirism in partner relationships.

In our survey of 200 volunteer college students, over half of the respondents (53%) met the criteria for either mild, moderate, or severe psychic vampirism in their relationships with either their partners or people in general. Eight percent met the criteria for severe psychic vampirism in their relationships with people in general. That percentage increased to twelve percent for severe psychic vampirism among college students in their relationships with their partners. Six percent of the respondents met the criteria for severe vampirism in their relationships with their partners as well as with people in general.

In our follow-on interviews, respondents who scored in the severe range of psychic vampirism with either their partners or people in general typically accepted the vampire nature of their interactions but rejected the epithet, psychic vampire, because they considered it a loaded term. Many of them presented a history of vampire-like interactions extending into their early teen years. They often volunteered that they knowingly extracted energy from others, including partners, acquaintances, and even strangers. A few of the respondents who scored in the severe range justified their vampirism by insisting that, while receiving energy in their vampire-like interactions, they also invested their own energy, especially in the early stages of building their romantic relationships. They conceded, however, that the energy transfer soon became one way, with themselves the sole recipient once the relationship was fully established.

The respondents in our survey often excused their behavior by noting the spin-off benefits of their vampire-like interactions. One respondent, who had a history of dermatitis, reported that prolonged absences from her partner always activated the disorder. She believed that she drew healthful energy from the interaction with her partner. Another respondent, who was in a body building program, admitted that he deliberately drew energy from other body builders, including his rivals in competitive events. His strategy included imagery of an in-coming flow of energy from his opponent.

Many of our respondents insisted that the energy they received through their vampire-like interactions was always put to good use. They were often high achievers who had clarified their career goals. Many of them were from affluent backgrounds, and highly active in extra-curricular affairs, including student government, athletics, and social organizations. Several of them had received recognition for their leadership roles, athletic achievements, and contributions to the college community.

Contrary to all reason, psychic vampirism occasionally involves the mutual consent of both vampire and victim. Consensual vampire relationships are typically characterized by a dominant partner who assumes the role of vampire. The weaker partner may see the vampire/victim interaction as a means of nurturing or saving the relationship; whereas the stronger partner often rationalizes the interaction as mutually satisfying.

Certain romantic relationships have the characteristics of consensual psychic vampirism, which we call the romantic vampire phenomenon. Our studies of this interesting phenomenon revealed several important gender features. Among college couples with admitted vampire elements in their relationships, the vampire was typically male. For older couples whose relationships included consentual vampire elements, the vampire was typically female. There is no easy explanation for these finding. They suggest that the college-age male and the older female have greater romantic vampire needs than either the younger female or older male. Other explanations focus on role expectations, with the older female expected to be more assertive in fulfilling her needs than either college-age females or males in general.

Although very little research data are available to show romantic vampire trends in partners with significant age differences of ten years or more, there is some evidence to suggest that the much older partner, whether male or female, in the consensual vampire relationship is more likely to assume the active role of vampire than the younger partner. Our studies of older vampires (age forty and above) noted that the older male vampire often sought a very young partner who, he believed, energized him with youth and vigor. The older female vampire appeared much less preoccupied with age differences in her partner selection.

Throughout our study of psychic vampirism, we used an objective, non-judgmental approach. Questionnaire results were interpreted in the context of other data, including interview results and observations of the aura. Our interviews with respondents who exhibited vampire-like characteristics always emphasized the developmental nature of human behavior and our innate capacity for change.

The Vampire Aura

Psychic vampirism as an adult adjustment style usually has a long history in which symptoms, along with related changes in the aura, often emerge in the early teen years. Faulty social learning and unfulfilled social needs are commonly present in the background of psychic vampires. Often because of limited opportunities for social interaction and comparison, psychic vampires develop their own patterns of social fulfillment. They begin early to exercise the energy receiving capacity of the aura. As the receiving functions of the aura become dominant over other aura characteristics, actual structural changes begin to occur in the visible aura.

Among the major aura characteristics signaling psychic vampirism are numerous voids and areas of washed-out or drab coloration along with a shadowy, external region. Among advanced psychic vampires, dark structures, sometimes called vampire tentacles, can be seen reaching beyond the area of normal aura activity. When preparing for interaction, the tentacles can be seen stretching outward as if in search of a host victim. Upon contact with the host, the tentacles either interface the aura for a slow absorption of energy, or they puncture the aura to draw instantly from its inner energy supply. The effects of the encounter are immediately visible in both the vampire and the host. As the host's aura recedes and diminishes in brightness, the vampire's aura expands and pulsates with new energy.

In our laboratory, we used electrophotography to investigate the effects of psychic vampirism on the human aura. For our research, we used the procedure to record the corona-discharge patterns around the right index fingerpad of professed psychic vampires and non-vampires. The shadowy, outer pattern, which we called the vampire shadow, was clearly visible in the photographs of vampires but never visible in the photographs of non-vampires. Visual inspection of the aura of our subjects confirmed the electrophotographic data. Figure 7 illustrates the distinguishing vampire shadow phenomenon. You will note the inner field of normal aura activity, and the surrounding outer field of vampire activity.

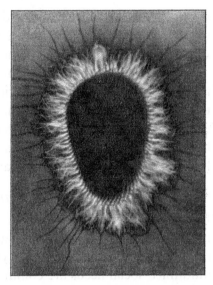

FIGURE 7. THE VAMPIRE SHADOW PHENOMENON. The darker outer region of activity signals psychic vampirism.

In the vampire attack, the outer field of activity expands to interact with the energy field of the host victim. Following the interaction, the vampire's inner field of activity assumes a remarkable but temporary glow, as indicated in Figures 8 and 9. In contrast, the host victim's energy field is markedly diminished in brightness and expansiveness following the attack, as illustrated in Figures 10 and 11 (see page 194). The effects of the vampire attack for both vampire and victim can last for several days.

The Finger Interlock Technique

Fortunately, we are not left defenseless in protecting ourselves against psychic vampire assaults on the aura. Procedures have been developed to prevent an attack and, when an assault is already underway, to promptly end it and prevent further loss of energy. Aura protection procedures, particularly those designed to terminate an attack, must be rapidly implemented. Since vampire attacks are usually brief—they may last only seconds—a quick response with immediate results

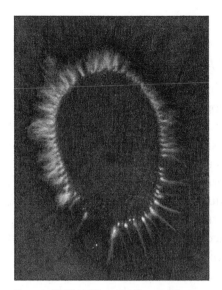 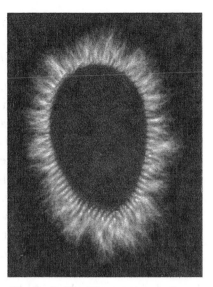

FIGURE 8. THE VAMPIRE *BEFORE* INFU-SION. Photo obtained before the attack illustrates the vampire's weak energy supply.

FIGURE 9. THE VAMPIRE *AFTER* INFU-SION. Photo obtained following the attack illustrates the vampire's new infusion of energy. Note the outer vampire shadow in both photographs.

is essential. The Finger Interlock Technique achieves that goal. It is an easily mastered procedure that can either prevent a vampire attack on the aura or instantly terminate it. Here is the procedure:

Step 1. Interlock Gesture. Immediately upon suspecting an imminent vampire attack (or if an attack is already underway), join the tips of the thumb and middle finger of each hand to form two circles. Then bring your hands together to form interlocking circles.

Step 2. Energy Protection. While maintaining the interlocked circles, close your eyes and envision a shield of powerful energy enveloping your total aura and effectively repelling any invasion of external forces.

Step 3. Energy Infusion. Envision the inner core of your energy system, pulsating with power and infusing your total being with abundant energy.

Step 4. Affirmation. Allow the infusion to reach its peak, then affirm: *My total being is infused with powerful energy. I am surrounded by a protective shield of power. I am safe and secure.*

In addition to preventing an imminent vampire attack or terminating an attack which is already in progress, the Finger Interlock Technique instantly energizes the aura and erects a protective outer shield, which we call the halo effect. The shield typically remains in place for several hours to effectively deflect other vampire invasion efforts. The effectiveness of the Finger Interlock Technique is illustrated by Figure 12 which includes before, and Figure 13 which includes after electrophotographs of the energy patterns around the right index finger. Note the halo effect with its accompanying infusion of energy following the Finger Interlock Technique.

The Finger Interlock Technique requires only seconds, and it can be used almost anywhere. Although it was designed to instantly repel

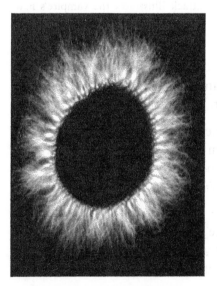

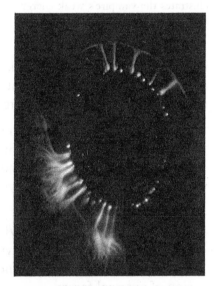

FIGURE 10. THE VICTIM *BEFORE* VAMPIRE ATTACK. Photograph obtained before the vampire attack illustrates the victim's normal energy supply.

FIGURE 11. THE VICTIM *AFTER* VAMPIRE ATTACK. Photograph obtained immediately after the attack illustrates the victims severe loss of energy.

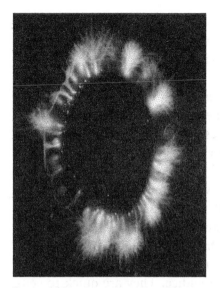

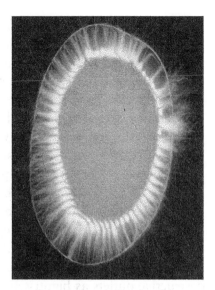

FIGURE 12. BEFORE INTERVENTION. Photo obtained *before* the Finger Interlock Technique depicts the loss of energy resulting from a psychic vampire attack.

FIGURE 13. THE HALO EFFECT. This photo illustrates the energizing infusion and halo effect resulting from the finger interlock technique.

the onslaught of vampirism, the technique can be used to energize and protect the aura from any negative invasion of external forces. It can be used to induce a relaxed, tranquil state, or to promote restful sleep. The procedure can be adapted to extinguish anxiety in such situations as job interviews and public presentations. Students find the technique particularly effective in reducing test anxiety and stimulating higher thought processes.

The Vampire Liberation Procedure

While considerable effort has been devoted to developing anti-vampire procedures, almost no attention has been given to ways of empowering psychic vampires to overcome their self-defeating vampire tendencies. Many professed psychic vampires are distressed by their compulsion to feed on the energies of others. Many of them attempt to break the chains of vampirism, only to discover that the addiction is beyond their control. Others repress their vampire drives, only to express them indirectly through other channels. With their tendencies buried in the subconscious, they may seek fulfillment through ostensibly unrelated activities, such as over-achievement, recognition, and humanitarian activities. They have been known to react to their suppressed tendencies by compulsive shopping, gambling, overeating, and substance abuse. They sometimes compensate for their perceived inadequacies by becoming overly involved in organizations and community activities. They may become religious extremists in their efforts to escape from themselves. As religious fundamentalists, they are often quick to condemn others who do not meet their standards or share their views. As suppressed vampires, they fit the Biblical description of the Pharisees and scribes who "make clean the outside of the cup and of the platter, but within they are full of extortion and excess." On a larger scale, they have been known to vent their suppressed vampire impulses through such destructive outlets as bigotry and prejudice. They are quick to censure groups and even boycott organizations that do not stoop to their levels of intolerance. Typically deficient in insight, they rationalize their behaviors and resist change until their subconscious vampire tactics utterly fail.

The essential conditions for overcoming vampirism in one's self are: (1) awareness of existing vampire tendencies and (2) a firm intent to change. The vampire must come to terms with the fact that only through commitment and concentrated effort can psychic vampirism, like any other disempowering behavior, by extinguished. Vampire tendencies must be recognized and accepted, not as vile and repulsive, but simply as unworkable. Self-blame and guilt, which can actually interfere with the empowerment process, are replaced with motivation and determination.

The Vampire Liberation Procedure was developed in our laboratory and tested for effectiveness among scores of admitted psychic vampires. The procedure was almost always effective except when the subject either resisted or was ambivalent about abandoning vampire interactions. The procedure requires an implementation plan which includes two practice sessions daily (upon awakening and at bedtime) over at least a two-week period and longer when necessary to eradicate vampire tendencies by activating new sources of energy. Here is the procedure:

Step 1. Solar Plexus/Fingertip Contact. Assume a comfortable, relaxed position, and rest the fingertips of both hands on your abdomen over the solar plexus region.

Step 2. Deep Breathing. Take in a deep breath and hold it as you count to three, then slowly exhale. Repeat the breathing exercise several times as your fingertips continue to rest on your abdomen.

Step 3. Energy Infusion. Close your eyes and envision your aura's innermost core situated in your solar plexus region as a powerful generator of abundant energy. Sense the energy generated by the aura's core as it radiates into your fingertips resting on your abdomen and spreads over your total body. Mentally unleash the energy blocked within yourself. Let your total being mentally, physically, and spiritually become fully energized. Allow the infusion process to continue until you are saturated and overflowing with energy.

Step 4. Cosmic Contact. Turn the palms of your hands upward and envision cosmic energy entering your hands and spreading through your total being, blending with your own energies and balancing them. Sense the accompanying attunement within your mind, body, and spirit.

Step 5. Self Affirmation. Join the tips of your fingers in a praying hands position and affirm: *I am filled and overflowing with abundant energy. Mentally, physically, and spiritually, I am attuned within my own being and with the universe. I am fully empowered in mind, body, and spirit. I will use the energies of my being to facilitate my own growth and to promote the well-being of people around me. I can generate abundant power within myself at any time by simply touching the tips of my fingers and affirming: I AM EMPOWERED!*

Step 6. Post-procedure Affirmation. To instantly activate at any time the empowering effects of this procedure, join the tips of your fingers and affirm: *I AM EMPOWERED!*

Summary

A major premise of psychic empowerment is an unfaltering belief in the human capacity, not only for change but for greatness. When growth is interrupted or our plans are derailed, the inner spark of greatness remains intact, a constant reminder of the immeasurable power available to each of us.

By tapping into the power within ourselves and the cosmos, we can discover the highest peak of human experience. Given abundant power, we can overcome any obstacle and meet every challenge. Nothing is impossible to the empowered mind, body, and spirit.

9

A Seven~Day Aura
Empowerment Plan

The loftiest edifices need the deepest foundations.

—George Santayana,
Winds of Doctrine
(1913)

A LL TOO OFTEN, the human aura has been seen simply as an external phenomenon with little relevance to our personal empowerment. The focus has been primarily on how to see and read the aura, with but slight attention devoted to its complex dynamics as a powerful force within a larger cosmic energy system. We now know that the observable aura is a powerful manifestation of an inner life force and the indestructible nature of our existence as a conscious being. Furthermore, we have found that the aura, with its inner core, is our link to the ultimate power of the cosmos. It is a powerhouse of potentials, but activating its powers, and more importantly, developing its capacities, requires a deliberate, concentrated plan of action.

The Seven-Day Aura Empowerment Plan is designed to initiate a totally new growth spiral that empowers us to reach a higher level of personal fulfillment. It includes several of the step-by-step strategies which we have previously discussed, and organizes them into a developmental plan that emphasizes our capacity for growth and change. The plan guides us toward a deeper understanding of the aura and its relevance to our personal empowerment.

Day One

Many important aura-related empowerment strategies require skill in viewing the aura. Developing your ability to view your own aura is one of the most important goals of our seven-day plan. Day one introduces four self-viewing strategies, each designed to facilitate viewing of the aura around the hand. Each procedure requires only a few seconds to bring the aura into clear view. For practice purpose, either natural or soft, indirect lighting with an off-white background screen is recommended for each procedure. You will find that viewing skills, once they are mastered, can be applied under almost any condition.

I. The Aura Hand-Viewing Procedure

Step 1. Relaxation. Let yourself become relaxed by taking in a few deep breaths and exhaling slowly as you clear your mind of all active thought.

Step 2. Finger Spread. Extend your hand, and hold it at arm's length with your fingers slightly spread against an off-white background.

Step 3. Visualization. Visualize a small dot floating in the space between your thumb and index finger.

Step 4. Fixed Gazing. Fixedly gaze at the imaginary dot until the aura appears, usually within seconds, first around your thumb and right index finger, then around your full hand and lower arm.

Step 5. Aura Viewing. Once the aura is clearly visible, shift your gaze directly to it, and observe its characteristics.

NOTE: Should you tire at any point in the exercise, take a few moments to relax, and then resume the procedure.

II. The Finger-Count Procedure

Step 1. Finger Count. With your hand outstretched and held with the fingers spread apart, slowly count your fingers one-by-one beginning with the thumb. Gaze briefly at the tip of each finger as you count it.

Step 2. Reverse Finger Count. As your hand remains outstretched and your fingers spread apart, reverse the counting procedure by slowing counting your fingers backward from five to one, beginning with the little finger and ending with the thumb. As in Step 1, gaze briefly at the tip of each finger as you count it.

Step 3. Finger Gaze. Gaze at the tip of your middle finger for a few moments, then expand your peripheral vision to include your full hand. Almost immediately, a soft white glow will appear around your hand, followed by the colorful aura.

Step 4. Aura Viewing. With the aura now in view, you can shift your attention directly to it and observe its features in detail.

III. The Hand Triangle Procedure
(Adapted for Self-Viewing)

Step 1. Triangle Formation. With your hands held at arm's length a short distance from the background screen, erect a triangle by first bringing together the tips of your thumbs to form the base of the triangle. Then bring the tips of your index fingers together to form the top of the triangle.

Step 2. Visualization. While viewing the triangle against the off-white screen, visualize a small dot at the center of the triangle and focus your full attention on the imaginary dot.

Step 3. Fixed Gazing. Fix your gaze on the imaginary dot and continue gazing at it until the aura appears, typically within seconds, first inside the triangle, and then around your hands and lower arms.

Step 4. Aura Viewing. Once the aura is visible, note its coloration, expansiveness, and other distinguishing features.

Step 5. Psychic Activation. To activate your psychic faculties, focus your full attention on the concentration of energy in the triangle formed by your hands as you allow psychic insight to unfold.

Step 6. Empowerment Affirmations. Conclude the procedure by affirming your power to view your own aura and use your aura energies as channels for psychic growth.

IV. The Palm-Motion Procedure

This strategy is designed to generate a transient but highly visible concentration of energy in the hands.

Step 1. Palm Contact. Bring the palms of your hands together lightly, and gently rub them against each other in first circular and then to-and-fro motions. You will notice almost immediately the build-up of warm energy in the palms.

Step 2. Palm Separation. With the palms of your hands remaining together, reach forward, and at arm's length, slowly separate your hands to create a narrow space between them. You will immediately notice a mild tingling in your palms and fingertips.

Step 3. Energy Perception. Center your attention on the narrow space between your hands, and note the whitish glow. Adjust the distance between your hands until color appears.

Step 4. Cupped Palms. With your hands still held at arm's length, gently cup your hands to create some distance between your palms while maintaining the narrow space between your fingertips.

Step 5. Energy Channel. After focusing for a few moments on the space between your fingertips, bring your fingertips together, and then slowly separate them. You will immediately see a channel of glowing energy between your fingertips.

Adjust the distance between your fingertips until you notice the appearance of color, which typically matches that of the color seen in the space between your hands in Step 3 above.

Step 6. Aura Viewing. Gaze at your cupped hands still facing each other until the aura appears around them, then turn your hands so that you face your palms. Note the enveloping aura and its various characteristics.

In Step 6 of this procedure, a ball of iridescent energy can often be seen gathering in the cupped hands.

Day Two

The activities of day two are centered on building your capacity to view the auras of other persons, a skill which is facilitated by your day-one practice of self-viewing activities. Three aura viewing procedures, each requiring a volunteer subject, are included, with several practice sessions recommended for each procedure. Although your will find that a single trial is usually sufficient to bring the aura into view, additional practice is usually necessary to fine-tune your viewing skills.

For each of the following procedures, either natural daylight or soft, indirect lighting is recommended, with the subject being viewed situated at distances of approximately ten feet from the viewer and approximately two feet away from an off-white, non-glossy background wall or screen. Each procedure requires only a few seconds to bring the aura into view.

I. The White-out Procedure

Step 1. Physical Relaxation. Give yourself permission to become physically relaxed through a simple, three-step technique called body scan: (1) With your eyes closed, mentally scan your body, beginning at your forehead and progressing downward. (2) Envision a soft glow of relaxation accompanying the scan and eventually enveloping your full body. (3) Silently affirm: *I am now fully relaxed.*

Step 2. White-out. Focus your eyes on your subject's forehead, and slowly expand your peripheral vision to encompass your subject's total surrounding. Once your peripheral vision reaches its limits, allow your eyes to fall slightly out of focus. You will then experience the "white-out effect," a phenomenon in which your subject's surroundings assume a milky-white glow.

Step 3. Focusing. Bring your eyes back into focus, and center your full attention on your subject's forehead. Almost immediately, the aura will come into view.

Step 4. Viewing. You are now ready to view the aura and focus your attention on its coloration and other characteristics. Should your eyes tire during viewing, close them for a few moments or look briefly into the distance away from your subject. If the aura begins to fade at any point during viewing, close your eyes briefly and then repeat the procedure.

II. The Triangle Erector Procedure

Step 1. Preliminaries. With the subject positioned approximately two feet from the background screen, designate the three points of a triangle by placing adhesive dots on the screen. One dot is placed a few inches above the subject, and two dots are placed at waist level, with one to each side of the subject at a few inches from the body.

Step 2. Pre-viewing Conditioning. At a viewing distance of approximately ten feet from your subject, conduct a body scan by closing your eyes for a few moments and mentally scanning your body from the head downward, releasing all tension as you go.

Step 3. Triangle Erector Exercise. Open your eyes and focus your full attention on the dot above your subject's head. After a brief moment of gazing at that point, shift your attention to the dot situated at your subjects lower left. Gaze at that point for a few moments, and then shift your attention to the dot at your subject's lower right. Following a brief moment of gazing at that point, complete the triangle by shifting your attention to your starting point—the dot above your subject. Continue gazing at that point until the aura comes into view, typically within a few seconds. Note: For some viewers, the aura will become visible early-on in the erection exercise.

Step 4. Aura Viewing. Shift your gaze from the dot above your subject and focus your attention directly on the aura. Note specific aura characteristics or areas of particular interest or activity. Should the aura begin to fade at any time during viewing, focus your attention on the dot above your subject and repeat the triangle erector exercise.

Step 5. Psychic Responsiveness. Note the psychic impressions, particularly clairvoyance, that often accompany this procedure.

NOTE: With practice, you will discover you can effectively substitute imaginary points for adhesive dots on the background screen.

III. The Hand Triangle Procedure

This procedure is effective for: (1) viewing the aura under relatively non-structured conditions and (2) generating relevant psychic impressions concerning the subject, especially precognition.

Step 1. Triangle Formation. Form a triangle with your hands by first bringing together the tips of your thumbs to form the base of the triangle. Then bring the tips of your index fingers together to form the top of the triangle.

Step 2. Frame Adjustment. Use the triangle as a frame within which to view your subject. Adjust the frame by moving your hands in and out until you find the distance which provides the ideal space within the triangle for viewing your subject.

Step 3. Aura Viewing. Observe your subject through the triangle until the aura appears, typically within seconds. Remove the triangle by slowly separating and then relaxing your hands. You can now view the aura in its fullness or focus on particular characteristics or areas of activity. Should the aura begin to fade, repeat the procedure.

Step 4. Psychic Responsiveness. Note the psychic impressions, particularly precognition, that often emerge spontaneously during the viewing process.

Day Three

The goal of day three is twofold: (1) To generate a fully energized mental, physical, and spiritual state through the Comprehensive Intervention Procedure, and (2) to generate a cosmically centered state within the self through the Cosmic Centering Procedure. Approximately thirty minutes should be allowed for each task.

I. The Comprehensive Intervention Procedure

This energizing procedure can be supplemented at Step 5 with imagery and affirmations related to specific goals, such as breaking unwanted habits, managing stress, or succeeding at an important task.

Step 1. Aura Pre-view. Find a quiet, comfortable place, and view your aura using any of the self-viewing procedures previously discussed.

Step 2. Body Scan. Settle back into a reclining or prone position, and clear your mind of all active thought. With your eyes closed, induce a deeply relaxed state by mentally scanning your physical body from the upper region down. Identify and release any accumulation of tension. Complete the body scan by taking in three deep breaths and exhaling slowly. Tell yourself after the third breath: *I am now fully relaxed.*

Step 3. Energizing Imagery. Envision a powerful glow emanating from deep within yourself and slowly infusing your total body with refreshing energy. Feel the warm, invigorating energy in your central body region gently spreading in all directions, enveloping your total body in a luminous glow of energy.

Step 4. Energy Infusion. Take a few moments to allow the infusion of powerful energy to reach its peak. Focus on particular body regions, such as specific joints or small muscle groups, and notice the deep infusion of energy. Should a point of weakness or tension remain, think of it as a discoloration, then promptly replace it with the revitalizing glow of energy.

Step 5. Affirmation. As your remain relaxed and energized, affirm: *My total being—mentally, spiritually, and physically—is fully infused with powerful, positive energy. I am enveloped in the light of love, peace, and power.* Specify your goals and envision them as realities. Affirm your power to succeed.

Step 6. Aura Post-view. Conclude the procedure by again viewing your aura using the same procedure you used in Step 1. Note the changes in your aura.

II. The Cosmic Centering Procedure

This procedure recognizes two major sources of power: One centered in the higher part of the self and the other centered in the higher part of the cosmos. Through cosmic centering, we can become intimately connected to both. The result is an empowered state of total inner and outer attunement. For this procedure, a reclining or prone position is recommended, with the legs uncrossed and hands resting comfortably to the sides.

Step 1. Aura Pre-view. View your aura using any of the self-viewing procedures detailed previously. Notice the specific features of your aura, including coloration, brightness, and expansiveness.

Step 2. Physical Relaxation. While resting comfortably, closed your eyes and focus only on your breathing. As you breathe deeply and rhythmically, let yourself become progressively relaxed. Take a few moments to envision a peaceful scene, such as a billowy cloud gently drifting in the breeze against a clear blue sky, and then affirm: *I am at peace with myself and the cosmos.*

Step 3. Inner Awareness. Center your full attention on the innermost part of your self. Visualize a luminous, inner core situated in your solar plexus. Think of it as an energy powerhouse radiating abundant energy that fuels your entire being—mental, physical, and spiritual.

Step 4. Energy Infusion. Notice the forceful infusion of resplendent energy. Visualize your body enveloped in a radiant glow, and affirm: *I am infused with powerful, radiant energy.*

Step 5. Cosmic Imagery. Envision the distant center of the cosmos as a brilliant core of powerful energy. Think of that core as the cosmic powerhouse that fuels the universe. Focus your full attention on its limitless power.

Step 6. Cosmic Empowerment. Picture a powerful channel of bright light connecting the luminous core of your inner being to the brilliant core of the outer cosmos. As you continue to picture the gleaming shaft of pure light, let yourself become fully infused with pure cosmic energy. Affirm: *I am attuned to the cosmos and empowered with abundant cosmic energy. I am fully energized and balanced mentally, physically, and spiritually.*

Step 7. Aura Post-view. Conclude the procedure by again viewing your aura, noting particularly any changes in coloration and intensity.

Day Four

Day four of our plan introduces two critical aura self-massage strategies. The X Self-massage is designed to enrich and expand the aura by distributing its energies more evenly. The Self-rejuvenating Massage revitalize the aura system and rejuvenates the underlying biological and psychological factors related to aging. Each procedure requires approximately thirty minutes and can be conducted in either the seated or reclining position with eyes closed.

I. The X Self-Massage

Step 1. The X Position. Begin the X Self-massage by closing your eyes (keeping them closed for the duration of the procedure) and crossing your arms to form an X across your chest. With your arms crossed and resting against your chest, place your hands on your shoulders as you breathe slowly, deeply, and regularly. Take a few moments to relax as you clear your mind of active thought.

Step 2. Aura Imagery. While maintaining the X position, envision your full aura, noting its colors, patterns, and unique features. Give particular attention to the aura surrounding your upper body.

Step 3. Two-stage Massage. *Stage I.* As your arms remain crossed, lift your hands and arms a few inches from your body, then gently stroke the aura around your chest and shoulders, using slow circular hand motions. Envision the aura around your hands and arms interacting with the aura around your chest and shoulders. Sense the energizing effects of the massage deep within your body.

Stage II. Uncross your arms and place your hands to the sides of your head, and with your palms turned toward your temples, use circular motions to gently massage the aura, being careful to avoid all physical touch. Extend the circular hand massage by moving slowly downward to include the shoulders, chest, abdomen, and hips. Further extend the massage by using brisk, vertical motions that sweep energies from your trunk region downward. Reverse the downward direction of the massage, slowing massaging upward with circular strokes, and finally culminating at the head region.

Step 4. Self-empowerment Affirmations. Return your arms to the original crossed position and, with your hands resting on your shoulders, affirm: *I am enveloped in positive, powerful energy. I am at my peak mentally, physically, and spiritually. I am empowered to achieve my highest goals.*

II. The Self-Rejuvenating Massage

Step 1. Relaxation. Slow your breathing and envision a vapor gently rising around you to envelop your total body. As the vapor slowly rises, let your body become increasingly relaxed. Affirm to yourself that the vapor signifies a higher cosmic energy force that empowers your physical body and aura system. Once your body is fully enveloped, allow the vapor to become transformed into a iridescent glow. Slowly breathe in the glow as your affirm: *I am absorbing peace and serenity throughout my total being.*

Step 2. Rejuvenation Regression. Mentally travel back in time, and envision yourself at your youthful prime, perhaps standing before a full length mirror, disrobed and glowing with the energies of youth. Note especially the radiant glow around your body and the youthful gleam in your eyes as you affirm: *This is the true me.* Focus your attention on your solar plexus region as the rejuvenating center of your aura system. Breath in the glow of youth surrounding your body, absorbing rejuvenating energy deeply within yourself. Affirm: *My total being is fully infused with rejuvenating energy.* Sense the energies of youth flowing throughout your body.

Step 3. Two-stage Rejuvenating Massage. *Stage I.* Massage the aura emanating from your central body region with slow, upward hand strokes that end with a gentle outward sweep. Focus first on the lower area and work your way upward using only vertical strokes and outward sweeps while always avoiding physical contact. Envision the energies related to aging as discolorations that are being swept away from your aura system. Upon reaching the head region, continue the upward vertical movements, but let them end with gentle backward strokes to the sides of your head. Conclude this stage of the massage with the upward facial sweep, a procedure that gently strokes the aura emanating from the face, using upward hand movements that end with a backward sweep over the head while envisioning a radiant glow of rejuvenating energy around the body.

Stage II. Rub your hands gently together as you visualize rejuvenating energy in the form of bright pink light being concentrated in your palms. Again massage your aura using the procedure as detailed in Stage I, beginning at your central body region and culminating with the face massage. Envision your aura as it takes on the pink glow of youth. As you stroke the aura around your face, notice the tingling, rejuvenating sensations. Allow the muscles in your face to respond to the upward strokes by soaking in rejuvenating energy.

Step 4. Concluding Affirmations and Post-massage Cue. The goal of this step is two-fold: first, to fortify the immediate results of the massage, and second, to establish the upward facial sweep as a post-massage cue for use on command to instantly activate rejuvenation. To achieve this goal, envision your body again enveloped in radiant energy as you affirm: *My total being is revitalized and infused with rejuvenation. I will, on command, instantly activate rejuvenation by upwardly stroking the energies emanating from my face as I envision the radiant glow surrounding my body.*

The upward facial sweep as a rejuvenation cue can be used almost anywhere and as often as needed. Frequent use of this rejuvenating gesture can generate a visible glow around the face while reducing or preventing the signs of aging, including neck and facial wrinkles.

Day Five

The activities of day five are based on our natural tendency to interact with nature, and the empowerment potential of those interactions. Two procedures are introduced to maximize that potential: The Empowerment Nature Walk and Tree Power Interaction.

I. The Empowerment Nature Walk

This procedure is designed to energize the aura while empowering us to achieve specifically designated personal goals through guided interactions with nature. While any safe natural setting is appropriate for the walk, a scenic vista or old-growth forest is recommended.

Step 1. Aura Preview. Before starting the walk, view your aura using any of the self-viewing techniques previously discussed.

Step 2. Goal Statement. Settle back and with your eyes closed, formulate your immediate goals and state them as specifically as possible. Ask yourself, "What do I hope to accomplish through this walk in nature?" Your goal may be simply to energize your aura system or to experience the sheer pleasure of the walk. On the other hand, you may want to overcome a certain growth blockage in your life, gain insight into yourself, find a solution to a particular problem, or resolve a personal conflict.

Step 3. The Walk. Select a safe, familiar place for walking. Walk at a comfortable pace, taking time to notice your surroundings. Think of the elements around you—plants, animals, rocks, and streams—as energized creations of nature with power to share. Let them speak to you as you absorb the vibrant energy gathering around you. Think of your surroundings as partners in your empowerment journey. Enjoy the miracles of life around you. Note your sense of oneness with nature, and tell yourself: *I am an integral part of all that exists.* Review your goals as formulated in Step 1, and affirm your power to achieve them.

Step 4. Reflection. At the end of the walk, look back on the experience and reflect on the interactions that occurred. Formulate detailed mental images related to the walk and file them away as snapshots in your mind for future reference. Review the empowering effects of the walk, then affirm: *I am empowered by this experience. By calling forth images related to it, I can at any moment unleash the flow of vibrant energy in my life.*

Step 5. Aura Post-view and Evaluation. View your aura again, using the same self-viewing technique as in Step 1, and note the changes. Re-affirm the empowering effects of the experience.

II. Tree Power Interaction

This is a structured, specialized procedure that utilizes the tree as a tangible, interactive object. Critical to the success of the procedure is the formulation of empowerment goals and the selection of a tree appropriate to those goals.

Step 1. Aura Viewing. View your aura, using any of the self-viewing procedures previously discussed. Note particularly the color, brightness, and magnitude of your aura.

Step 2. Goal Statement. Formulate your goal(s) for the interaction. Your goal may be to infuse your aura with healthful energy, energize a dormant region in your energy system, add color to the aura, correct an energy dysfunction, or illuminate the total aura, to list but a few of the possibilities. Other goals not directly related to the aura can involve an unlimited range of personal concerns, including physical, emotional, social, career, and so forth.

Step 3. Tree Selection. Selecting a tree initiates the interactive process. It is important to select a tree that appeals to you personally and seems appropriate for your particular goals. It can be a familiar tree or one that you notice for the first time. It can be either isolated or closely surrounded by other trees. Once you select a tree, note your sense of connection to it. Before approaching the tree, interact with it by observing its unique characteristics such as height, proportions, and structure. Mentally engage the tree as a receptive partner in your empowerment efforts. Acknowledge the tree as a magnificent creation of nature with an abundant supply of energy.

Step 4. Tree Power Infusion. As you approach the tree, sense its surrounding field of energy interacting with your own energy field. Touch the tree first with your fingertips, thereby connecting the antennae of your body to the tree as the powerful antenna of the earth. Note the wondrous infusion of cosmic energy permeating your total energy system. Rest your palms against the tree and note an even greater infusion of intense power. Your total being is now linked not only to the tree, but to the limitless power of the cosmos.

Step 5. Tree Power Interaction. With your palms resting against the tree, visualize your aura system interacting with the energy system of the tree. Sense the powerful changes occurring in your aura system, from its outer edges to its innermost core. Gently stroke the tree, and let the tree speak to you. Reaffirm your connection to the infinite power of the cosmos.

Step 6. Reflection. Disengage the tree and bring your hands together in a praying hands position. Reflect on the powerful interaction experience. Look upward at the tree as you review your empowerment goals. Address the tree and affirm your goals as present realities. For instance, if your goal is to energize your aura, affirm: *I am totally infused mentally, physically, and spiritually with abundant energy,* as you envision your aura glowing with bright energy. If your goal is better health, affirm: *I am now fully infused with healthful energy.* If your goal is to quit smoking, affirm: *I am now smoke-free.* Even goals concerning the distant future can be stated as present realities. If you are a student and your goal is future career success, affirm: *Career success is my destiny.* Accompany your affirmations with goal-related imagery to further strengthen the empowering effects of the procedure.

Step 7. Aura post-view and Evaluation. View your aura and compare it to your earlier viewing. Note the changes, particular in coloration, brightness, and magnitude.

Following the procedure, periodically reflecting on the experience as images of the tree are formed can instantly reactivate the procedure's empowerment results.

Day Six

Two critical activities—the Moon Power Strategy and the Star Power Strategy—are introduced in day six of our plan. Through the Moon Power Strategy, you can introduce important changes in your aura's color and structure, depending on the nature of your goals. The strategy requires the full moon as a tangible tool, or when the moon is absent, imagery of the moon. Through the Star Power Strategy, you can generate an inner state of complete cosmic attunement. The strategy introduces a star as our link to the cosmic dimension of our existence. Frequent use of these strategies increases their empowerment effectiveness.

I. The Moon Power Strategy

Step 1. Initial Aura Viewing. View your aura using any of the full-aura viewing techniques discussed in Chapter 3. Pay particular attention to the aura's coloration and intervention needs.

Step 2. Goal Formulation. Specifically state your aura intervention goals, and then affirm: *I will use this procedure to achieve these goals.*

Step 3. Moon Viewing. View the full moon, or when the moon is absent, form a mental picture of it. Allow the image of the moon to become firmly fixed in your mind.

Step 4. Moon Imagery. With your eyes closed, envision the full moon and focus your full attention on it. Exclude all other images from your mind. Allow sufficient time for the moon to vividly appear.

Step 5. Empowerment Activity. With the full moon image firmly fixed in your mind, recall each of your goals and engage the moon as your empowerment partner. If your goal is to infuse your aura with brightness, envision the moon as radiating bright energy and your total aura system absorbing it. If your goal is to add a particular color to a designated area in your aura, envision the moon taking on that color and transferring it either as moon beams or as a sphere of color to your aura, infusing the designated area with new energy. If your goal is to introduce a new rim of color into your aura, envision the moon changing to that color and dispersing it as bright energy to your full aura.

Step 6. Final Aura Viewing. View your aura again, using the same viewing procedure as in Step 1. Note the changes in your aura. Conclude the exercise with the simple affirmation: *I am fully empowered.*

II. The Star Power Strategy

Step 1. Body Scan. Settle back, take in a few deep breaths, and let your mind become passive by clearing it of active thought. With your mind emptied of problems, mentally scan your physical body, beginning at the upper region and progressing slowly downward. Note any build-up of tension and mentally release it.

Step 2. Aura Scan. This step requires three mental scans of the aura—the energy scan, color scan, and structural scan. With your eyes closed, envision the full aura enveloping your physical body. Then, beginning above your head, slowly scan your aura downward as you sense its energy frequencies. Note any disruption or interference in energy patterns. Having completed the energy scan, conduct a color scan, again beginning at the aura's uppermost region and progressing slowly downward. Allow images of the aura's color make-up to accompany the scan, including regions and enveloping layers of color as well as areas of discoloration. Finally, conduct a structural scan of the aura beginning again at the aura's uppermost region. Note particular structural features, paying special attention to possible dysfunctions, such as voids, breaks, or fissures.

Step 3. Star View. Scan the night sky and select a certain star for viewing. If a star is not visible, form a mental image of one. Focus your full attention on the star, whether real or imagined, and sense your personal connection to it. Give the star a name—any name that comes to mind—and address the star as your intimate link to the cosmos. Think of it as a miniature but powerful replica of the cosmic core. Imagine the star connected to the center of the cosmos by a beam of light and endowed with the same limitless power as the cosmic core.

Step 4. Power Draw. Envision your aura and a beam of light connecting it to the star. Visualize bright cosmic energy from the star progressively infusing your aura system, beginning at your aura's upper region and gradually moving downward. Sense the pulsating energy as it fills your aura, infusing voids and repairing dysfunctional or damaged regions. Sense the harmonious vibrations within your aura as it becomes filled with vibrant cosmic energy.

Step 5. Final Aura Scan. As you sense pulsating cosmic energy infusing your aura system, mentally scan your aura from its upper region downward. Note its vibrancy, balance, and attunement. Sense harmonious frequencies throughout your aura system. You are now attuned to the innermost core of your being and to the powerful core of the cosmos.

Step 6. Conclusion. Conclude the exercise with the simple assertion: *My total being is infused and empowered with pure cosmic energy.*

Day Seven

Our aura empowerment plan would be incomplete in the absence of strategies that effectively protect the aura from assault. A central theme of our plan is building a strong aura system, which is our best defense against any potentially disempowering force around us, including the so-called psychic vampire. But since even the strongest aura can come under siege, we need a practical, efficient strategy to either prevent an assault, or if an assault is already underway, to promptly end it. The Finger Interlock Technique achieves that goal by instantly energizing the aura and erecting a protective outer shield, called *the halo effect,* which typically remains in place for several hours to deflect other assault efforts.

Step 1. Interlock Gesture. Immediately upon suspecting an imminent attack on the aura (or if an attack is already underway), join the tips of the thumb and middle finger of each hand to form two circles. Then bring your hands together to form interlocking circles.

Step 2. Energy Protection. While maintaining the interlocked circles, close your eyes and envision a shield of powerful energy enveloping your total aura and effectively repelling any invasion of external forces.

Step 3. Energy Infusion. Envision the inner core of your energy system, pulsating with power and infusing your total being with abundant energy.

Step 4. Affirmation. Allow the infusion to reach its peak, then affirm: *My total being is infused with powerful energy. I am surrounded by a protective shield of power. I am safe and secure.*

The Finger Interlock Technique requires only seconds, and it can be used almost anywhere. Aside from energizing and protecting the aura, it can be used to induce relaxation and a serene mental state, build self-confidence, and stimulate our highest thought processes. With practice, simply forming the finger interlock (Step 1) is sufficient to instantly activate the empowerment effects of the procedure.

Conclusion

We began our study of the human aura with a goal statement: to explore the basic nature and makeup of the aura and second, to develop relevant strategies that utilize the aura, not simply as a resource, but as our link to the cosmic source of our existence. Throughout this book, our pursuit of that goal has been steadfastly self-empowerment oriented. We have discovered an able aura specialist residing in each of us, a specialist with power to see the aura, interpret it, intervene into its functions, and most important of all, utilize it as an interactive energy system in ways that promote our mental, physical, and spiritual well-being.

Yet, in retrospect, we admittedly have barely scratched the surface of this magnificent, inexhaustible phenomenon. We have uncovered only a few of the possibilities, but hopefully we have opened the door for many new, exciting discoveries. As we rocket into the new century, our toughest challenge lies within ourselves—developing our highest capacities and applying them to empower our lives. Once committed to the task, we can, individually and globally, reach our destiny for greatness.

Glossary

Amethyst Power Strategy. An aura empowerment strategy that uses the amethyst as a tool to unleash health and fitness energy while balancing the aura system.

Astral Projection. See *out-of-body experience.*

Astral Travel. See *out-of-body experience.*

Aura Body-building Massage. A specialized aura massage strategy designed to remediate specific aura deficiencies and energize particular functions or affected areas.

Aura Caress. A hands-on procedure designed to assess the aura's frequency level.

Aura Color Massage. A specialized aura massage strategy designed to enrich the aura's coloration or add totally new colors to the aura.

Aura Dowsing Procedure. An assessment and diagnostic strategy using dowsing to analyze the aura's immediate and external design.

Aura Elasticity Massage. A specialized aura massage strategy designed to generate sufficient flexibility in the aura to close voids and restore the aura's normal energy functions.

Aura Hand-viewing Procedure. An aura self-viewing procedure using finger-spread and visualization to bring the aura surrounding the hand and lower arm into view.

Aura Map and Analysis Form. A form used for recording the results of aura dowsing.

Aura Massage. An energy interaction between the subject and a massage specialist who uses hand-massage techniques to empower the aura.

Aura Power Tools. Tangible tools that can be used to empower the aura.

Aura Repair Strategy. A specialized aura massage strategy designed to repair the damaged aura, particularly when fissures or points of darkness are present.

Aura Scan. A procedure in which the aura is mentally scanned, typically from the upper region downward.

Aura Self-healing Massage. A specialized massage procedure designed to introduce new healing energies into the physical body, and whenever needed, to restore normal functions to specific organs and systems.

Aura Self-massage. Any of several specialized massage procedures designed to promote self-interaction with the aura in order to activate the aura's highest empowerment capacities.

Aura Signature. The constellation of characteristics that provide a reasonably stable representation of an individual's aura.

Birth Number. A single digit value representing the date of an individual's birth.

Body Scan. A procedure in which the physical body is mentally scanned, typically from the head down, to release tension and induce a deeply relaxed state.

clairvoyance. The psychic perception of objects, conditions, situations, or events.

Color Transfer. An aura empowerment procedure designed to maximize the effects of Crystal Programming by using the same programmed crystal to enrich the aura with additional energy related to specific empowerment goals.

Comprehensive Intervention Procedure. A self-empowerment strategy that uses physical relaxation, mental imagery, and positive affirmations to energize the aura.

corona-discharge photography. See *electrophotography*.

Cosmic Centering Procedure. An aura intervention strategy designed to empower the aura by connecting the self to the higher cosmic sources of power.

cosmic congruency. A condition of total oneness in which the individual experiences balance within the self and an intimate connection to the universe.

cosmic genotype. The cosmic make-up which ensures the uniqueness of each individual as a spiritual entity; the cosmic counterpart of biological genotype.

Crystal Programming. A step-by-step procedure designed to program the crystal through a two-way interaction with the crystal and the careful input of appropriate goal-related components.

Crystal Scan. A crystal selection procedure that takes into consideration the quality of our interactions with the crystal, and the nature of our empowerment goals.

4-D Formula. An aura empowerment strategy utilizing the pyramid model as a tool to balance and attune not only the aura but the total person.

dowsing. A procedure using rods to access psychic information.

electrophotography. A photographic procedure which generates a corona-discharge around a specimen which is then recorded on film. Also known as *Kirlian photography* and *corona-discharge photography*.

Emerald Rejuvenation Procedure. An age-management approach designed to link the emerald's rejuvenation properties to the power within ourselves to influence the normal aging process.

Empowerment Nature Walk. A structured procedure designed to energize the aura and empower us to achieve specifically designated personal goals through guided interactions with nature.

ESP. See *extrasensory perception.*

extrasensory perception (ESP). The knowledge of, or response to, events, conditions, and situations independently of known sensory mechanisms or processes.

Finger-Count Procedure. An aura self-viewing strategy that requires counting the fingers of the out-stretched hand to bring the aura into view.

Finger Interlock Technique. A aura self-protection procedure that either prevents a psychic vampire attack or instantly terminates it.

Finger-Spread Method. A self-hypnosis induction and aura empowerment procedure in which the aura is viewed and the PK faculty is activated to empower the aura.

Focal-Point Procedure. An aura viewing strategy that requires focusing on a shiny object positioned on a screen behind the subject.

General Aura Massage. An aura massage procedure designed to unleash new energy into the aura while setting the stage for more specialized massage strategies.

halo effect. A protective outer shield erected around the aura through the Finger Interlock Technique. See *Finger Interlock Technique.*

Hand Triangle Procedure. An aura viewing strategy in which the thumbs and index fingers form a triangle through which the subject is viewed. The procedure can be adapted for self-viewing.

hypnosis. A trance state in which receptivity to suggestion is heightened.

Interaction Questionnaire I. A questionnaire designed to assess psychic vampire tendencies in one's relationship to people in general.

Interaction Questionnaire II. A questionnaire designed to assess psychic vampire tendencies in one's relationship to a particular partner.

interdimensional materialization. A phenomenon in which discarnate energy appears in visible form.

Kirlian photography. See *electrophotography*.

Luminous Massage. A specialized aura massage strategy designed to infuse the total aura system with brightness and abundant energy.

Moon Power Strategy. An aura empowerment procedure that uses the full moon, or an image of it, as a tangible tool for inducing change in the aura system.

NDE. See *near-death experience*.

near-death experience (NDE). An experience in which death appears imminent, often accompanied by a sense of separation of consciousness from the biological body.

numerology. The study of numbers and their significance beyond the expression of quantity.

OBE. See *out-of-body experience*.

out-of-body experience (OBE). A state of awareness in which the locus of perception shifts, resulting in a conscious sense of being in a spatial location away from the physical body. Also known as *astral travel* and *astral projection*.

Pain Intensity Scale. A scale used in pain management to assess the intensity of pain.

Pain Management Aura Massage. A specialized strategy designed to reduce or eliminate pain and replace it with healing energy.

Palm-Motion Procedure. An aura self-viewing strategy designed to generate a transient but highly visible concentration of energy in the hands.

Peripheral Glow Method. A self-hypnosis induction and aura empowerment procedure in which the aura is viewed and intervention measures are implemented.

phantom leaf effect. In electrophotography, a relatively rare phenomenon in which the energy pattern enveloping a full leaf remains intact after a part of the leaf is removed.

PK. See *psychokinesis.*

precognition. The psychic awareness of the future.

Psychic Perception Procedure. A strategy designed to facilitate aura viewing independent of sensory perception.

Psychic Self-perception procedure. An aura self-viewing strategy designed to expand self-awareness of the aura by activating inner psychic faculties.

psychic vampire. An individual who practices psychic vampirism. See *psychic vampirism.*

psychic vampirism. A phenomenon in which the underdeveloped aura system with deficient energy resources habitually invades the aura systems of others and draws energy from them.

psychokinesis (PK). The capacity of the mind to influence objects, events, and processes in apparent absence of intervening physical energy or intermediary instrumentation.

Pyramid of Power. A procedure using the pyramid model as a tool to energize, expand, and empower the total aura system.

romantic vampire phenomenon. A romantic relationship which has the characteristics of consensual psychic vampirism.

Sapphire Star Procedure. An empowerment procedure using the sapphire to induce cosmic attunement and balance within the self.

self-hypnosis. A self-induced trance state in which receptivity to one's own suggestions is heightened.

Self-rejuvenating Massage. A specialized self-massage procedure designed to either slow or reverse aging by activating the aura's rejuvenating energies and channeling them to designated targets.

shadow phenomenon. The shadowy, outer pattern seen in the corona-discharge photographs of psychic vampires.

Specialized Aura Massage. Any aura massage strategy designed to empower a particular aura function or remediate a particular aura deficiency or dysfunction.

spherical therapy. A procedure using the paranormal manifestation of a sphere of apparent healing energy.

Star Power Strategy. An aura empowerment strategy that uses a star as an empowerment tool to generate a state of complete cosmic attunement.

subliminal perception. The perception of and response to stimuli at levels below the conscious thresholds for perception.

Subliminal Perception Technique. An aura viewing technique designed to bring subliminal perceptions of the aura into conscious awareness.

table tilting. A group procedure that employs a small table to initiate interaction and access information, particularly of discarnate significance.

telepathy. The sending and receiving of cognitive and affective contents.

third eye. A mental faculty associated with clairvoyance and remote viewing.

Tree Power Interaction. A structured, specialized procedure that uses the tree as a tangible, interactive object to empower the aura.

Triangle Erector Procedure. An aura viewing strategy requiring the mental erection of a triangle using designated points on a screen situated behind the subject.

vampire aura. An aura pattern characterized by dark tentacles reaching beyond the area of normal aura activity.

Vampire Liberation Procedure. A procedure designed to liberate the psychic vampire from vampire tendencies and behaviors.

vampire tentacles. Among psychic vampires, dark structures that reach beyond the area of normal aura activity.

Walk-in Procedure. An interactive aura viewing strategy that progressively guides the viewer into the subject's energy zones until the aura becomes visible.

white-out effect. A short-lived optical effect characterized by an expansive, milky-white visual field surrounding a point of focus. See White-out Procedure.

White-out Procedure. An aura viewing strategy which requires expanding peripheral vision to induce an optical effect that precedes the appearance of the aura. See *white-out effect.*

X Massage. A self energizing aura massage procedure designed to stimulate the aura system and distribute its energies more evenly throughout the aura.

Suggested Reading

Andrews, T. *How to See and Read the Aura*.St. Paul: Llewellyn Publications, 1993.

Antonovsky, A. *Health, Stress, and Coping*. San Francisco: Josey-Bass, 1979.

Bagnall, O. *The Origins and Properties of the Human Aura*. New York: University Books, 1970.

Baruss, I. *The Personal Nature of Notions of Consciousness*. New York: University Press of America, 1990.

Becker, E. *The Denial of Death*. New York: Free Press, 1973.

Bergin, A. E., & Garfield, S., eds. *Handbook of Psychotherapy and Behavior Change*. New York: Wiley, 1994.

Bowers, B. *What Color is Your Aura?* New York: Pocket Books, 1989.

Butler, W. E. *How to Read the Aura*. Wellingborough: Aquarian Press, 1971.

Cayce, E. *Auras*. Virginia Beach: A.R.E. Press, 1945.

Claxton, G. *Noises from the Darkroom: The Science and Mystery of the Mind*. London: Aquarian/Harper Collins, 1994.

Crabtree, B. F., & Miller, W. L., eds. *Doing Creative Research.* Newbury Park, CA: Sage, 1992.

d'Aquili, E. G., & Newburg, A. B. *Consciousness and the Machine.* Zygon, 1996, pp. 31, 235-252.

Dennett, D. C. *Consciousness Explained.* Boston: Little, Brown, 1991.

Fordor, N. *Handbook of Psychic Science.* New York: University Books, 1966.

Gergen, K. J. *Toward Transformation in Social Knowledge.* New York: Springer-Verlag, 1985.

Godel, K. *Collected Works (Vol. 2).* New York: Oxford Press, 1990.

Held, B. S. *Back to Reality.* New York: Norton, 1995.

Jones, A. *Seven Mansions of Color.* Marina del Rey, CA: DeVorss & Co, 1982.

Joy, W. B. *Joy's Way.* Boston: Houghton Mifflin, 1979.

Leder, D. *The Absent Body.* Chicago: University of Chicago Press, 1990.

Lewis, R. *Color and the Edgar Cayce Readings.* Virginia Beach, VA: A.R.E. Press, 1973.

Merleau-Ponty, M. *The Phenomenology of Perception.* New York: Routledge, 1962.

Nelson, T. O. *Consciousness and metacognition.* American Psychologist, 1996, pp. 51, 102-115.

Ostram, J. *Understanding Auras.* London: Harper Collins, 1993.

Ostrander, S. & Schroeder, L. *Psychic Discoveries Behind the Iron Curtain.* New York: Bantam Books, 1971.

———. *Handbook of Psi Discoveries.* London: Sphere Books Limited, 1977.

Panchadasi, S. *The Human Aura*. Chicago: Yoga Publication Society, 1950.

Powell, A. E. *The Etheric Double*. Wheaton, IL: Theosophical Publishing House, 1983.

Schultz, D. P., & Schultz, S. E. *A History of Modern Psychology* (6th ed.). Fort Worth, TX: Harcourt Brace, 1996.

Slate, J. *Investigations into Kirlian Photography: Final Technical Report*. Huntsville: U. S. Army Missile Research and Development Command, 1977.

————. *The Kirlian Connection: Final Technical Report*. New York: Parapsychology Foundation, 1985.

————. *Psychic Phenomena: New Principles, Techniques and Applications*. Jefferson, NC: McFarland, 1988.

————. *Self-Empowerment: Strategies for Success*. Bessemer, AL: Colonial, 1991.

————. *Psychic Empowerment: A 7-Day Plan for Self-Development*. St. Paul: Llewellyn Publications, 1994.

————. *Psychic Empowerment for Health and Fitness*. St. Paul: Llewellyn Publications, 1996.

————. *Astral Projection and Psychic Empowerment*. St. Paul: Llewellyn Publications, 1997.

Taylor, S. E. *Positive Illusions: Creative Self-deception and the Healthy Mind*. New York: Basic Books, 1989.

————. *Health Psychology* (3rd ed.). New York: McGraw-Hill, 1995.

Index

A

B

C

D

E

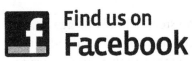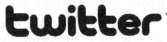
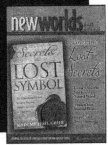

ANCIENT TEACHINGS FOR BEIGNNERS

Douglas DeLong

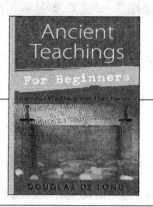

Uncover hidden knowledge from the mystery schools of ages past. This book is designed to awaken or enhance your psychic abilities in a very quick and profound manner. Rather than taking years to achieve this state, you will notice results within a few short weeks, if not instantly. Explore hidden secrets of the ancient mystery schools as you progress through each chapter, from opening your third eye and crown chakras to seeing and reading the human aura.

1-56718-214-3, 384 pp., 5 ³⁄₁₆ x 8, illus. $13.95

WRITE YOUR OWN MAGIC
The Hidden Power in Your Words

RICHARD WEBSTER

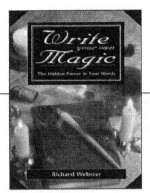

Write your innermost dreams and watch them come true!
This book will show you how to use the incredible power of words
to create the life that you have always dreamed about. We all have
desires, hopes and wishes. Sadly, many people think theirs are unrealistic or unattainable. *Write Your Own Magic* shows you how to
harness these thoughts by putting them to paper.

Once a dream is captured in writing it becomes a goal, and your
subconscious mind will find ways to make it happen. From getting a
date for Saturday night to discovering your purpose in life, you can
achieve your goals, both small and large. You will also learn how
to speed up the entire process by making a ceremony out of telling
the universe what it is you want. With the simple instructions in this
book, you can send your energies out into the world and magnetize
all that is happiness, success, and fulfillment to you.

0-7387-0001-0, 5 ³⁄₁₆ x 8, 312 pp. $13.95

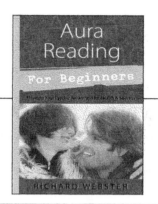

AURA READING
FOR BEGINNERS
Develop Your Psychic Awareness
for Health & Success
RICHARD WEBSTER

When you lose your temper, don't be surprised if a dirty red haze suddenly appears around you. If you do something magnanimous, your aura will expand. Now you can learn to see the energy that emanates off yourself and other people through the proven methods taught by Richard Webster in his psychic training classes.

Learn to feel the aura, see the colors in it, and interpret what those colors mean. Explore the chakra system, and how to restore balance to chakras that are over- or under-stimulated. Then you can begin to imprint your desires into your aura to attract what you want in your life. These proven methods for seeing the aura will help you:

- Interpret the meanings of colors in the aura
- Find a career that is best suited for you
- Relate better to the people you meet and deal with
- Enjoy excellent health
- Discover areas of your life that you need to work on
- Make aura portraits with pastels or colored pencils
- Discover the signs of impending ill health, drug abuse, and pain
- Change the state of your aura and stimulate specific chakras through music, crystals, color

1-56718-798-6, 208 pp., 5 ³/₁₆ x 8, illus. $12.95

SELF-HYPNOSIS
FOR A BETTER LIFE

WILLIAM W. HEWITT

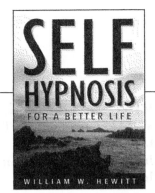

The sound of your own voice is an incredibly powerful tool for speaking to and reprogramming your subconscious. Now, for the first time, you can select your own self-hypnosis script and record it yourself. *Self-Hypnosis for a Better Life* gives the exact wording for 23 unique situations that can be successfully handled with self-hypnosis. Each script is complete in itself and only takes 30 minutes to record. You simply read the script aloud into a tape recorder, then replay the finished tape back to yourself and reap the rewards of self-hypnosis!

Whether you want to eradicate negativity from your life, attract a special romantic partner, solve a problem, be more successful at work, or simply relax, you will find a number of tapes to suit your needs. Become your own hypnotherapist as you design your own self-improvement program, and you can make anything happen.

1-56718-358-1, 256 pp., 5 ³/₁₆ x 8, illus., softcover $11.95

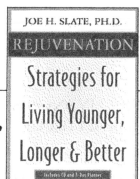

JOE H. SLATE, PH.D.

REJUVENATION

Strategies for
Living Younger,
Longer & Better

Includes CD and 7-Day Planner

REJUVENATION:
STRATEGIES FOR LIVING YOUNGER,
LONGER & BETTER
Includes CD with meditations & exercises
JOE H. SLATE, PH.D

Preventing mutations that cause illness, keeping artery walls open and free of blockage, and prolonging the ability of cells to reproduce are reasonable expectations for anyone willing to develop his or her capacity for rejuvenation and longevity. Whatever your current age, you possess the built-in potential to repair and recreate yourself. This book offers forty-five new rejuvenation strategies, many of which were developed in a college laboratory setting. By protecting and fortifying your innermost energy system, you can slow the aging process and even reverse its effects in some instances. Aging factors are flexible and responsive to deliberate intervention. When you turbocharge your inner age-defying mechanisms, you can slow the winged chariot of time and live a longer, richer life.

- Learn the Fourteen Golden Rules for Rejuvenation and eight strategies for thwarting the effects of negative stress
- Energize biological systems and influence brain activity through self-hypnosis
- Transcend biological boundaries by cultivating connections with higher cosmic energy and dimensions
- Connect with the creative power of the universe through interactions with nature

1-56718-633-5, 240 pp., 6 x 9 $19.95

To order, call 1-877-NEW WRLD
Prices subject to change without notice

THE HEALER'S MANUAL
A Beginner's Guide to Energy Therapies

TED ANDREWS

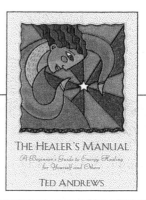

THE HEALER'S MANUAL

A Beginner's Guide to Energy Healing for Yourself and Others

TED ANDREWS

Did you know that a certain Mozart symphony can ease digestion problems...that swelling often indicates being stuck in outworn patterns...that breathing pink is good for skin conditions and loneliness? Most dis-ease stems from a metaphysical base. While we are constantly being exposed to viruses and bacteria, it is our unbalanced or blocked emotions, attitudes and thoughts that deplete our natural physical energies and make us more susceptible to "catching a cold" or manifesting some other physical problem.

Healing, as approached in *The Healer's Manual*, involves locating and removing energy blockages wherever they occur—physical or otherwise. This book is an easy guide to simple vibrational healing therapies that anyone can learn to apply to restore homeostasis to their body's energy system. By employing sound, color, fragrance, etheric touch and flower/gem elixers, you can participate actively within the healing of your body and the opening of higher perceptions. You will discover that you can heal more aspects of your life than you ever thought possible.

0-87542-007-9, 256 pp., 6 x 9, illus., softcover $14.95

To order, call 1-877-NEW-WRLD
Prices subject to change without notice

AURAS:
See Them in Only 60 Seconds!

MARK SMITH

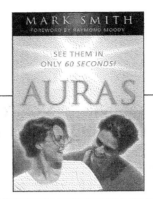

Your aura is the physical manifestation of your soul. You are already aware of this electro-magnetic energy, which is responsible for the good or bad "vibes" you get from other people. The aura's brightness, color and clarity denote various stages of peace, wellness and happiness. Science can measure it and even photograph it. The most astonishing fact of all is that anyone can learn to see auras in 60 seconds or less. This is the first book to show you how.

When you improve your auric vision, you can actually see illness or disease in the aura before it manifests in the body. Once you master the basic techniques, you can use breathing and meditation to stabilize and increase your own auric energy. This book also reveals the auras of luminaries such as Jackie Onassis; Jerry Garcia; James Taylor; Al Gore, Sr.; and others.

1-56718-643-2, 168 pp., 6 x 9, softcover $13.95

To order, call 1-877-NEW-WRLD
Prices subject to change without notice

CONNECTING TO THE POWER OF NATURE

Joe Slate

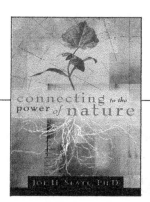

From the calming grace of a garden to the stabilizing strength of a tree, nature holds a magnificent power—one that awakens human potential. *Connecting to the Power of Nature* opens a gateway to self-discovery, helping you achieve an attuned, balanced, and empowered state of mind, body, and spirit. This unique book offers an extensive collection of enjoyable and inspiring step-by-step activities and meditations, using rocks, trees, flowers, leaves, and other natural elements. Cope with grief, manage stress, get insight into problems, discover new power in yourself, and accomplish your goals by tapping into nature's power. The possibilities for creating a richer and more rewarding life are endless.

0-7387-1566-2, 216 pp., 5³⁄₁₆ x 8, softcover $14.95

To order, call 1-877-NEW-WRLD
Prices subject to change without notice

PRACTICAL GUIDE TO CREATIVE VISUALIZATION
Proven Techniques to Shape Your Destiny

DENNING & PHILLIPS

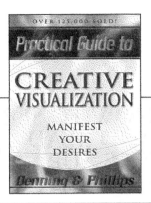

All things you will ever want must have their start in your mind. The average person uses very little of the full creative power that is his, potentially. It's like the power locked in the atom—it's all there, but you have to learn to release it and apply it constructively.

IF YOU CAN SEE IT...in your Mind's Eye...you will have it! It's true: you can have whatever you want, but there are "laws" to mental creation that must be followed. The power of the mind is not limited to, nor limited by, the material world. *Creative Visualization* enables humans to reach beyond, into the invisible world of Astral and Spiritual Forces.

Some people apply this innate power without actually knowing what they are doing, and achieve great success and happiness; most people, however, use this same power, again unknowingly, incorrectly, and experience bad luck, failure, or at best an unfulfilled life. This book changes that. Through an easy series of step-by-step, progressive exercises, your mind is applied to bring desire into realization! Wealth, power, success, happiness even psychic powers...even what we call magickal power and spiritual attainment...all can be yours. You can easily develop this completely natural power, and correctly apply it, for your immediate and practical benefit. Illustrated with unique, "puts-you-into-the-picture" visualization aids.

0-87542-183-0, 294 pp., 5¼ x 8, illus., softcover $12.95

To order, call 1-877-NEW WRLD
Prices subject to change without notice

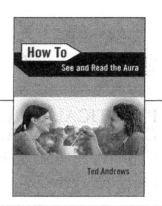

SPIRIT GUIDES &
ANGEL GUARDIANS
Contact Your Invisible Helpers

RICHARD WEBSTER

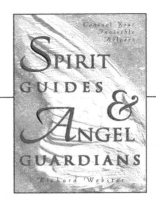

They come to our aid when we least expect it, and they disappear as soon as their work is done. Invisible helpers are available to all of us; in fact, we all regularly receive messages from our guardian angels and spirit guides but usually fail to recognize them. This book will help you to realize when this occurs. And when you carry out the exercises provided, you will be able to communicate freely with both your guardian angels and spirit guides.

You will see your spiritual and personal growth take a huge leap forward as soon as you welcome your angels and guides into your life. This book contains numerous case studies that show how angels have touched the lives of others, just like yourself. Experience more fun, happiness and fulfillment than ever before. Other people will also notice the difference as you become calmer, more relaxed and more loving than ever before.

- Find your life's purpose through your guardian angel
- Use time-tested methods to contact your spirit guides
- Use your spirit guides to help you release negative emotions
- Call on specific guides for nurturing, support, fun, motivation, wisdom
- Visit your guides through past-life regression

1-56718-795-1, 368 pp., 5 ³/₁₆ x 8, softcover $12.95

To order, call 1-877-NEW-WRLD
Prices subject to change without notice

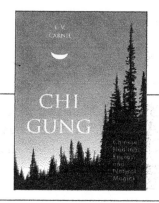